THE BOOK OF

Diabetic
Cooking

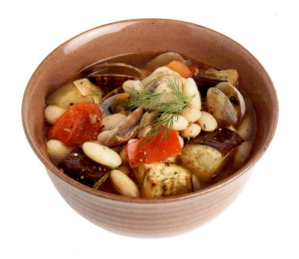

THE BOOK OF
Diabetic
Cooking

Jeanette Parsons Egan, M.S., R.D.

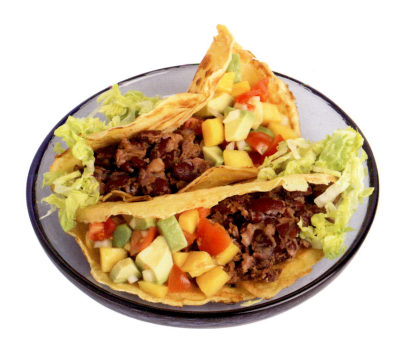

HPBooks

HPBooks
A member of Penguin Group (USA) Inc.
375 Hudson Street, New York, New York 10014, USA
Penguin Group (Canada), 10 Alcorn Avenue, Toronto,
Ontario M4V 3B2, Canada (a division of Pearson Penguin
Canada Inc.)
Penguin Books Ltd., 80 Strand, London WC2R 0RL, England
Penguin Group Ireland, 25 St. Stephen's Green, Dublin 2,
Ireland (a division of Penguin Books Ltd.)
Penguin Group (Australia), 250 Camberwell Road,
Camberwell, Victoria 3124, Australia (a division of Pearson
Australia Group Pty. Ltd.)
Penguin Books India Pvt. Ltd., 11 Community Centre,
Panchsheel Park, New Delhi—110 017, India
Penguin Group (NZ), cnr. Airborne and Rosedale Roads,
Albany, Auckland 1310, New Zealand (a division of Pearson
New Zealand Ltd.)
Penguin Books (South Africa) (Pty.) Ltd., 24 Sturdee Avenue,
Rosebank, Johannesburg 2196, South Africa
Penguin Books Ltd., Registered Offices: 80 Strand, London
WC2R 0RL, England

An imprint of Chrysalis Books Group plc

Photographer: Philip Wilkins
Home Economist and Stylist: Mandy Phipps
Editor: Katherine Edelston
Designer: Cara Hamilton
Production: Don Campaniello
Filmset and reproduction by: Anorax Imaging Ltd

ISBN: 1-55788-469-2

PRINTING HISTORY
HPBooks trade paperback edition / August 2005

Notice: The information contained in this book is true and
complete to the best of our knowledge. All recommendations
are made without any guarantees on the part of the author or
the publisher. The author and publisher disclaim all liability in
connection with the use of this information.

Printed and bound in China

10 9 8 7 6 5 4 3 2 1

CONTENTS

INTRODUCTION

THE STATISTICS

Diabetes is a rapidly growing worldwide problem. In the United States, the American Diabetes Association estimates that there are currently over 18 million people with diabetes. In Canada there are 2 million individuals with diabetes and in the United Kingdom there are over 1.7 million. The World Health Organization (WHO) has targeted diabetes as a major threat to global public health, because of the infrastructure and financial resources needed to treat the disease. WHO estimates that by 2030, the number of people with diabetes will have doubled.

WHAT IS DIABETES?

Diabetes mellitus, usually called diabetes, is a condition in which there is an inability of the body to produce or use insulin, which is a hormone produced by the pancreas necessary for the utilization of glucose. Glucose (along with other nutrients) is produced when the foods we eat are broken down into simpler units in our digestive tract and is the body's main source of energy. Glucose cannot be used unless insulin is present to move it from the blood into the cells. If the levels of blood glucose (blood sugar) increase above normal, the result is high blood sugar. There are two basic types of diabetes: type 1 and type 2.

Type 1 diabetes
Type 1 is the less common type, found in probably less than 10 percent of all diabetics. It is caused by a complete or almost complete lack of insulin production by the pancreas. It has sometimes been called juvenile-onset diabetes, because it often develops during childhood but can strike at any age. In order for individuals with type 1 to control their diabetes insulin must be administered. Diet and exercise also play important roles in maintaining normal blood glucose levels and preventing the complications associated with diabetes.

Type 2 diabetes
Type 2 diabetes, the most prevalent type, is caused by either low insulin production or the body's inability to use it (insulin resistance). Type 2 is often developed in midlife, thus it is also referred to as adult-onset diabetes. Recently there has been an alarming increase in the number of adolescents and even children who are diagnosed with type 2 diabetes, as well as an increase in the number of adults with the disease. Type 2 diabetes is often associated with excessive weight gain and reduced physical activity. A few individuals with type 2 diabetes can control their condition with diet and exercise alone, with weight loss for those who are overweight. Some people require oral glucose-lowering medications (see pages 8–9) and even insulin if they cannot achieve a normal blood glucose level with diet and exercise.

Gestational diabetes
There is a third type of diabetes that is usually temporary—gestational diabetes. It develops during the last stages of pregnancy. Women with gestational diabetes need to work closely with their health care providers concerning diet, exercise, and medications. With gestational diabetes there is a risk of miscarriage, excessively large babies, or even stillbirths. Women who experience gestational diabetes are also at risk of developing either type 1 or 2 diabetes later in life.

WHO GETS DIABETES?

The risk factors for developing type 1 diabetes are less established but include genetic, autoimmune, and environmental factors. It sometimes develops following a viral illness. There are several well-defined risk factors for type 2 diabetes. They include a family history of diabetes, being over 40 years of age, being overweight, a member of an ethnic group with an increased risk, and previous abnormal glucose tolerance test. Anyone who is obese should be tested for diabetes, including children and adolescents.

WHAT ARE THE SYMPTOMS OF DIABETES?

Although some individuals with diabetes show no symptoms, most experience some of the following: increased thirst, dry mouth, frequent skin, gum, or bladder infections, cuts and bruises that are slow to heal, numbness or tingling in hands and feet, fatigue, and frequent urination. Anyone experiencing these symptoms should consult with his or her physician.

WHAT ARE THE SIDE EFFECTS OF DIABETES?

Complications of poorly controlled diabetes include heart disease and stroke, high blood pressure, blindness, kidney disease, nervous system diseases, amputation of limbs, dental disease, and pregnancy complications. According to the U.S. Center for Disease Control, those with diabetes are likely to experience the following complications when compared to those without the condition: two to four times higher risk of death from heart disease, two to four times higher risk of stroke, increase in nervous system damage affecting various organs, higher incidence of gum disease, infectious diseases, stillbirths, and high blood pressure. The risk of death is about two times that of people without diabetes. It is also the major cause of blindness. Tight control of blood glucose levels can decrease the risk of complications by half.

CONTROLLING DIABETES

Some of those with type 2 diabetes can initially control their condition

Below: *When planning meals, include a variety of dark green and orange vegetables which are rich in vitamins and antioxidants.*

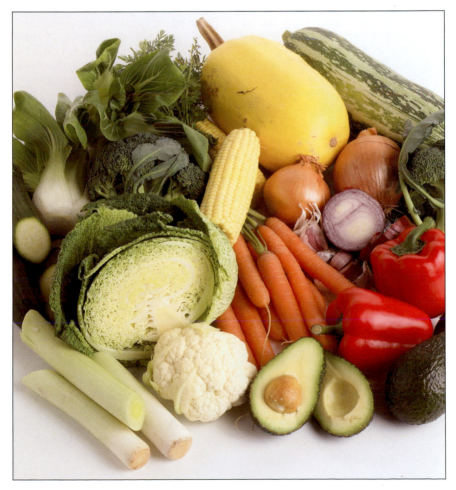

with diet and exercise alone. For those who are overweight, a gradual reduction in body weight is usually the first step.

Diet

Those with diabetes should eat a healthful diet by choosing a variety of foods. In general these foods should be low in saturated fat and dietary cholesterol and high in fiber. Because of the risk of high blood pressure, the amount of sodium should be limited. It is important for those with diabetes to eat the correct amount of calories to maintain a reasonable weight. Dietary intake should help maintain near-normal blood glucose levels, and help prevent complications, such as heart disease by maintaining favorable blood cholesterol and triglyceride levels. For children with diabetes, food intake must allow for normal growth and development and be modified as needed to account for physical activity.

If overweight, losing as little as 10 percent of total body weight can often be enough to return blood glucose to near normal levels. Weight loss is often beneficial for those with heart disease, lowering levels of cholesterol and triglycerides and reducing blood pressure.

General dietary guidelines
- Choose foods low in saturated fats; saturated fat intake should be less than 10 percent of total calorie consumption per day.

Below: Try to eat whole grain breads and cereals, nuts, and fruits every day, because they are good sources of vitamins, minerals, fiber, and good fats.

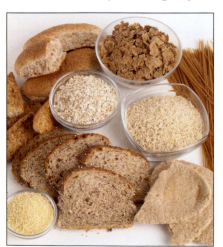

- Limit total fat intake to about 30 percent of total calories.
- Select a calorie level that will maintain a reasonable body weight or aid in slowly reaching a reasonable weight.
- On average, consume 300 mg or less of cholesterol per day.
- Include a fish meal at least once week. Fatty fish, such as salmon and sardines, are high in good fats, omega 3 fatty acids, which help protect against heart disease.
- Choose complex carbohydrate foods over ones containing mostly sugar. Sugar can be eaten, but high-sugar foods often contain empty calories.
- Eat a high-fiber diet, about 30 g of fiber per day for adults.
- Limit the amount of salt (sodium).
- Choose foods high in antioxidants—red, orange, deep-yellow, and dark-green vegetables, such as kale, broccoli, spinach, and tomatoes; fruits, such as berries, plums, and cherries; and tea.

Exercise

In addition to helping control diabetes by aiding in weight loss, exercise has a direct effect on blood glucose levels by reducing insulin resistance. Anyone with diabetes who wants to start an exercise program should consult his or her health care provider before beginning. Exercise also has positive benefits on heart health by reducing levels of cholesterol and triglycerides and reducing blood pressure.

Oral glucose-lowering medications

Oral medications work by either stimulating the pancreas to produce

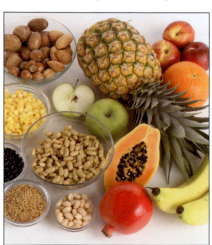

more insulin, reducing the amount of glucose produced by the liver, decreasing the cell's resistance to insulin, or by delaying the absorption of glucose from the small intestine into the blood or by a combination of these actions. Individuals who are on glucose-lowering medications often take more than one kind. The current medications are divided into the following five classes:

Alpha glycosidase inhibitors delay the absorption of glucose.
Biguanide reduces the amount of glucose produced by the liver and decreases insulin resistance.
Meglitinides stimulate the pancreas' to increase insulin production in surges, producing insulin peaks.
Sulfonylureas stimulate the pancreas to make insulin.
Thiazolidinediones reduce insulin resistance.

Insulin
Insulin is available in quick, intermediate, and slow acting forms or in combinations of slow and intermediate acting insulin. Some individuals with diabetes use an insulin pump for insulin delivery and others inject insulin, sometimes several times a day. Oral insulin tablets and inhaled insulin are currently being studied as alternative ways to deliver insulin.

Glucose monitoring
An important part of managing or controlling diabetes is glucose monitoring. This is a useful aid in determining if the health plan developed by you and your health care professional is working. Most individuals with diabetes do this several times a day by pricking a finger and putting a tiny drop of blood on a test strip that is read by a glucose monitor or meter. It is important to keep a record of your blood glucose values so you can discuss them during your next visit with your health care provider. Follow the advice of your health care professional when deciding how often to check your blood glucose. One important reason for checking blood glucose values is to prevent hypoglycemia (low blood sugar), especially in those taking insulin or some of the oral medications.

In addition to daily checks at home, there is another test, the A1C, that is performed two to three times each year, depending on how well blood glucose levels are controlled. It measures the amount of glucose attached to hemoglobin in the blood. The finger prick test indicates what the glucose level is at the time of the test, but the A1C records how well the glucose levels have been controlled over the past three months.

NUTRITION 101

The foods we eat are composed of carbohydrates, protein, fats, and other essential nutrients such as minerals and vitamins. Of these only the carbohydrates, protein, and fats (along with any alcohol we consume) contain calories. Carbohydrates and protein contain the same amount of calories, and fats twice as much for the same weight, with alcohol in between.

Carbs, Carbs, Carbs
Carbohydrates are divided into two groups: simple carbohydrates, such as sugars (see more about sugars and sweeteners, page 13), and complex carbohydrates, starches and fiber. Sources of carbohydrates include grains, fruits, and starchy vegetables. With the emphasis on low-carb diets, some may think that all carbohydrates are the same and should never be eaten. This is not the case. Carbohydrate-containing foods such as fruits are excellent sources of vitamins, minerals, and antioxidants. Whole grain foods such as breads and cereals supply B vitamins and minerals and are a good source of fiber. Choosing the right carbohydrate-rich food is important.

What is dietary fiber and why is it important?
Dietary fiber is a component of complex carbohydrates. Fiber comes only from plants; there is none in meats. Fiber is not digested in the small intestine, where most foods are broken down, but passes unchanged into the large intestine. There are two types of fiber, soluble and insoluble, and they work differently in the body. Most plants contain both types.

Soluble fiber includes pectins, beta glucans, gums, and psyllium (sometimes used as a laxative). Because soluble fiber dissolves in water, it can form gels when cooked and in the intestinal tract. These gels slow the passage of food through the digestive system and help moderate glucose absorption, preventing a sharp increase in blood glucose after eating. Soluble fibers may also bind to bile acids in the small intestine, preventing their absorption. The liver converts cholesterol to bile acids and preventing their absorption forces the liver to produce more, therefore reducing the overall supply of cholesterol in the body.

Most insoluble fiber is cellulose, but it also includes lignins and hemicellulose. Insoluble fiber is important for a healthy digestive tract—it keeps everything moving along. It does this by absorbing water and keeping the contents of the bowel soft, enabling the muscles in the walls of the intestine to function without creating too much pressure. Excess pressure causes the formation of small pouches called diverticula, which can become inflamed. Lack of fiber in the diet can cause constipation and hemorrhoids. High-fiber foods may be protective in the prevention of one of the common cancers, that of the colon.

Foods high in fiber are more satisfying because they take longer to digest and can decrease overall food consumption. They also give a sense of fullness in the stomach. In addition, most high-fiber foods are low in calories.

How much fiber is enough?

About 30 g of fiber a day is probably the right amount for most adults. This is about twice the estimated current intake. Fiber intake should be increased slowly to prevent stomach upsets and flatulence. It is very important to have adequate fluid intake on a high-fiber diet, as much as two quarts each day.

Ways to increase fiber intake and good carbs

- Eat the skins of fruits and vegetables. Rinse them with warm water or use a fruit and vegetable wash and gently scrub with a vegetable brush and rinse thoroughly. Choose organic foods when available.
- Substitute whole fruits for fruit juices.
- Choose high-fiber cereals and oatmeal for breakfast and use them in baked goods.

- Add beans and other legumes to your diet. If you use canned beans, choose low-sodium or no-salt added ones. If these are not available, drain and rinse canned beans to remove some of the sodium. You can also cook extra dried beans when you have the time and freeze them to use later.
- Choose a tablespoon of nuts or some popcorn for a snack.
- Eat more vegetables, including raw ones, in soups, salads, and other dishes.
- Remember that dried fruit is high in fiber but also high in sugar.
- Eat cooked green soybeans (edamame) as a snack.
- Choose whole grain foods such as pasta and breads rather than "white" ones. Whole grain or whole-wheat should be listed first on the ingredient list.
- Eat barley, bulgur, and other whole or minimally processed grains, the less processed the grain the more fiber and bran it contains.
- Add unprocessed wheat bran to meat loaves and casseroles.
- Substitute a small amount of oat bran for some of the flour in baking.
- Eat red, blue, and purple berries, either fresh or frozen without sugar, for their fiber and antioxidants.

Glycemic Index

The glycemic index (GI) rates foods according to how much they raise blood glucose levels after eating. While the glycemic index provides general information on how individual foods may affect food glucose levels, it does not indicate what happens when a complete meal composed of several foods are eaten. However, it is an indication of what foods to select when planning meals.

Protein

About 15 to 20 percent of your calories should come from protein. In general, persons with diabetes should choose protein foods that are low in saturated fat and cholesterol to reduce the risk of heart disease. Remember that cholesterol comes only from animals—there is none in plants. Protein is needed for growth in children and adolescents and for maintenance in adults. Three ounces of cooked meat or 1 cup cooked

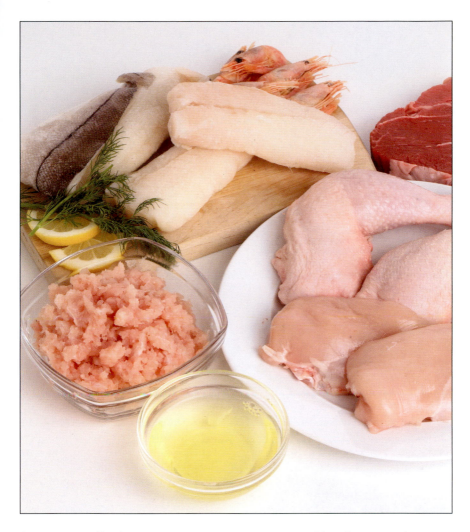

Above: Good low-fat protein choices include seafood, chicken, and lean trimmed meats, such as beef round.

beans is usually the correct amount for one adult serving.

Good low-fat animal protein sources
- Lean meat, such as pork tenderloin, beef round, flank steak, and extra-lean ground beef and pork
- White meat of chicken and turkey, including extra-lean ground turkey, without the skin
- Fish and shellfish
- Egg whites
- Fat-free or reduced-fat dairy foods

Good vegetarian protein sources
- Tofu, available in regular and low-fat versions
- Soybeans and other dried beans, peas, and lentils
- Nuts, including nut butters

GOOD FAT, BAD FAT

The amount and type of fat in the diet is important; high-fat foods are high-calorie foods. Fats should make up no more than 30 percent of daily calories. There are three types of fat: saturated, polyunsaturated, and monounsaturated and many foods contain some of each. The majority of fat in the diet should be monounsaturated fat. Saturated fat—butter, cheese, bacon, coconut, and palm, should make up less than 10 percent of total calories. Saturated fats tend to increase serum cholesterol levels, especially LDL (bad) cholesterol, which is a risk factor for heart disease. Monounsaturated fats increase the level of HDL (good) cholesterol and polyunsaturated fats reduce both good and bad cholesterol.

FOODS HIGH IN MONOUNSATURATED FATS

- Almonds
- Avocados
- Canola oil

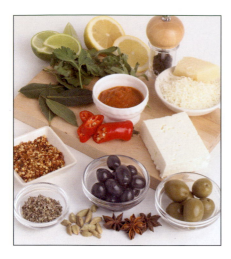

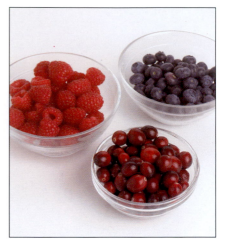

Above (left and right): Fruits and vegetables supply vitamins, minerals, fiber, and antioxidants, all of which are important in a healthy diet.

- Cashews
- Natural peanut butter, peanuts, and peanut oil
- Olives and olive oil
- Pecans
- Sesame seeds and sesame oil

Trans fats
When unsaturated fats such as oils that are liquid are changed into solid form, the position of the fatty acids change from the normally *cis* to the *trans* form. This is of concern because trans fatty acids seem to increase the LDL (bad) cholesterol in much the same way that saturated fat does.

Ways to reduce fat intake
- Choose lower-fat versions of favorite foods. Most reduced-fat foods have a better flavor and are more satisfying than fat-free foods, which often have added sugars, and may have the same amount or even more calories than the standard product.
- Use less fat at the table, such as on toast or added to a baked potato.
- Use nonstick cookware, which requires less fat.
- Try cooking spray for sautéing vegetables or coating foods for roasting.
- Use less fat in cooking. Steam, bake, roast, or poach foods instead of frying.
- Choose leaner cuts of meats, such as pork tenderloin or extra-lean ground beef.
- Replace sauces high in egg yolks and butter with lighter ones.

- Reduce portion size. Choose a trimmed 4-oz steak or $1/2$ cup of a starchy food.
- When choosing dairy products, use ones made from skim or reduced-fat milk.
- Use high-fat foods, such as olives and cheeses, as flavoring agents rather than the main ingredient.
- Use egg whites, liquid egg substitutes, low-fat tofu, or pureed low-fat cottage or ricotta cheese to replace some of the egg yolks in cooking.
- Read food labels and compare amounts of fat.

SODIUM

Over two-thirds of those with diabetes in the U.S. have blood pressure above normal levels. High sodium intake can increase the blood pressure in some individuals. For this reason limiting salt intake is often recommended to reduce the risk.

Ways to reduce sodium intake
- Use herbs, spices, and citrus juices to season food without adding salt.
- Read food labels and compare products to get ones lower in sodium. Choose no-salt added or reduced-sodium canned foods.
- Use fresh vegetables or vegetables frozen without salt.
- Choose minimally processed foods.
- Limit the use of condiments, such as pickles and olives, and commercial sauces.
- Reduce the intake of processed meats, such as cold cuts and hot dogs.
- Always taste food before adding salt at the table.

HOW SWEET IT IS

Sweetening agents can be divided into those that supply calories and noncaloric ones that supply less than 5 calories per serving. They are sometimes called nutritive (with calories) or nonnutritive (without calories).

Sweeteners that contain calories
Sugar (table sugar or sucrose) was once banned from diabetic diets, but research indicates that it does not raise blood glucose levels any more than other carbohydrates. However it is suggested that its use be limited, because high-sugar foods are often high in fat and contain empty calories (without important nutrients). In cooking, particularly in baked goods, sugar does more than add sweetness. It enhances flavors, aids in browning, and adds structure to the food. Often the amount of sugar can be reduced by about one-third without affecting the baked product.

Fructose is about one-third sweeter than sucrose (most sugars end in "ose") and can be used in cooking. Use one-third less than regular sugar in recipes. Fructose does not seem to raise glucose levels as much as sucrose but large amounts may increase LDL (bad) cholesterol levels.

Liquid sweeteners—molasses, honey, corn syrup, maple syrup, sorghum, and fruit juices, all contain sugars and are counted as carbohydrates in the diet.

Sugar alcohols (polyols)—mannitol, sorbitol, xylitol, lactitol, isomalt, maltitol, and hydrogenated starch hydrolysates (HSH), contain half to one-third less calories than sugar. They are often used in sugar-free candies and other products. Many sugar-free gums are sweetened with sugar alcohols because they do not cause dental caries. Because these sugars are less sweet than sucrose, more must be used to get the sweetness of sugar; this can mean that a product could contain enough sugar alcohol to contribute a significant amount of carbohydrate and may have an effect on blood glucose levels. If consumed in large amounts some of them can have a laxative effect and can cause cramping.

Is sugar-free really free?
Foods that are labeled sugar-free are not necessarily carbohydrate-free if they contain sugar alcohols. Even if these types of foods do not contain sugar or other carbohydrates they may still be high in fat and calories. In general, it is best not to assume that just because a product is labeled sugar-free or is marketed to those with diabetes that it can be freely consumed.

Sweeteners without calories
These are sometimes called artificial sweeteners or sugar substitutes, but their correct names are noncaloric or nonnutritive sweeteners. There are five noncaloric sweeteners approved for use in the U.S. by the Food and Drug Administration (FDA). These are aspartame, acesulfame-K, neotame, saccharin, and sucralose. (Cyclamate is not approved for use in the U.S. but is used in the U.K. and neotame is approved for the U.S. but not the U.K.)

Aspartame is roughly 200 times sweeter than sugar. Because it is made of two amino acids, it is digested as a protein (which contain 4 calories per gram). It can be used in cooking but is not heat stable at higher temperatures. It is sold as Equal® and used in manufactured foods as Nutrasweet®. Sugar Lite™ from Equal® is a blend of Equal® and sugar.
Acesulfame potassium (or acesulfame-K) is about 200 times sweeter than sugar. It is heat stable and can be used in cooking and baking. It is sold as Sunett®, Sweet & Safe®, and Sweet One®.
Neotame may be as much as 7,000 times sweeter than sugar. Approved for use by the FDA in 2002, it is not available yet. It has been used in New Zealand and Australia.
Saccharin is 200 to 700 times sweeter than sugar. It has a slightly bitter or metallic aftertaste. It is sold as Sweet and Low®, Sweet Twin®, Sweet 'N Low® Brown, and Necta Sweet®.
Sucralose is 600 times sweeter than sugar. Stable in heat and cold, it can be used in baking and cooking and in chilled desserts, such as ice creams. It is marketed as Splenda® and Splenda Granular®. Splenda® Sugar Blend for Baking is a blend of Splenda® and sugar.

Cooking with noncaloric sweeteners
Each of the available noncaloric sweeteners varies in chemical makeup and how they react when used in food preparation. The ones that are heat stable can be used in cooking and baking. They are best used in foods such as custards and stirred puddings that do not rely on sugar for browning and to provide bulk and texture to the final product. Some sweeteners tend to mask flavors and the sweet taste lingers in the mouth. Others may add a too sweet taste, even when used in recommended amounts, or impart a flavor of their own. Experiment with different products to determine which one works best for you.

The sugar/noncaloric sweetener combinations can be used much like sugar in cooking, because a high percentage of the product is sugar. It is one way to obtain a standard baked good with less sugar. An easy way to learn more about using a specific product is to visit the manufacturer's

Below: A few well-chosen pieces of equipment, such as good nonstick pans, make cooking easier and cleanup faster.

website for recipes and useful tips on using the products.

EQUIPMENT AND TOOLS: A STEAMY SUBJECT

There are some pieces of equipment and tools that will make it easier to prepare foods without using a lot of fat. Because cooking with fresh and whole foods requires more time, the right piece of equipment or tool will make the work go more quickly and efficiently.

Nonstick cookware should be good quality, because heavy pans will cook more evenly without burning. It is best to use low or medium temperatures when cooking with nonstick pans, and they should never be placed empty over high heat. Regular baking pans can also be lined with parchment paper.

An indoor electric grill or an outdoor gas or charcoal grill can be used to cook fish, meats, poultry, and vegetables. The fats drain away from the meat and poultry as they cook and the high heat adds crispness and

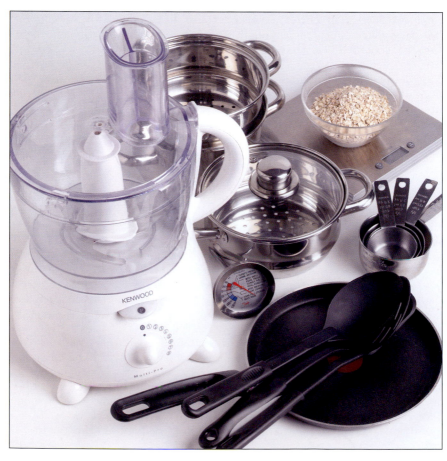

flavor without the need for a sauce. If a grill is not available, the broiler unit of your oven can substitute, but the flavor is not quite as good.

A steamer pot is a good investment or you can use a steamer insert in a large saucepan or Dutch oven for steaming vegetables or seafood.

A blender and/or a food processor aids in pureeing sauces, fruits, and vegetables, pureeing tofu to use in cooking, and for making smoothies.

A kitchen scale is helpful in measuring ingredients and in determining portion size.

A strainer is useful for rinsing canned beans to remove excess salt, draining pasta, and for rinsing fresh vegetables and fruits.

Heat-resistant silicone spatulas and spoons are favorite kitchen helpers for stirring sauces, vegetables, and for mixing. They can be used to stir boiling mixtures without melting and they will not scratch nonstick surfaces. Regular spatulas will melt when used for cooking.

Measuring cups and spoons are necessary to accurately measure ingredients.

Kitchen timers and instant-read thermometers are important when preparing lean meats and poultry to avoid overcooking, which results in tough meat, or undercooking, which might be a food safety issue.

Sharp knives and cutting boards make food preparation easier, especially if you are trying to use more fresh ingredients instead of canned or frozen ones.

ABOUT THE RECIPES

Cholesterol and saturated fats: The amount of cholesterol in the recipes was reduced by substituting egg whites or tofu for eggs in cooking and in breakfast dishes. Low-fat dairy products were used whenever possible to cut the amount of saturated fats and cholesterol. Lean meats and poultry cuts were selected for the main dishes.

Fats: Olive oil, canola oil, and sesame oil, all high in monounsaturated fats, were used in preparing the recipes. The fat content of many of the recipes can be lowered further by "sautéing" the onions and other seasoning in vegetable or chicken broth or water or by using cooking spray. No-trans fats margarine was used in a few of the recipes.

Fiber: Whole grain flours and cereals were used in baked goods. Fresh vegetables and fruits were used throughout the book. Cooked (or canned) dried beans were added to salads, soups, and main dishes.

Sodium: An effort was made in reducing the sodium content of recipes by using no-salt, reduced-sodium, or light products when they were available. Most recipes are seasoned to taste so the final amount of sodium and salt is up to the cook.

Sweeteners: Both sugar and a noncaloric sweetener (Splenda®) were used. When sugar was used to sweeten, it was less than that used in standard recipes. Some recipes used a combination of sugar and Splenda®.

NUTRITIONAL ANALYSIS

The nutrients in the recipes were calculated using the Food Processor® for Windows Nutrition & Fitness software program, version 7.8, by esha RESEARCH. Optional ingredients in the recipes were not included in the analysis. Ingredients that did not have a specific amount or were to taste were not analyzed. The first number was used when there was a range in ingredients or in the number of servings, such as 1–2 cups or 4–6 servings.

The recommendations and recipes in this book are general guidelines based on available information and should not be used to replace instructions provided to patients with diabetes by health care professionals such as physicians, diabetes educators, or registered dietitians. Always consult your health care professional before making any changes in diet, exercise habits, or medications.

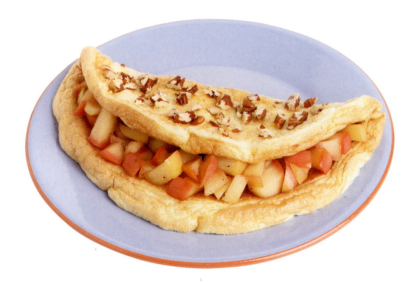

APPLE-FILLED OMELET

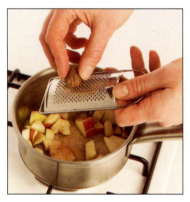

2 egg whites
1 egg
1/4 teaspoon salt
freshly ground pepper, to taste
1 tablespoon freshly grated Parmesan cheese
FILLING:
1/2 apple, cored and diced
1 teaspoon brown sugar
dash each of ground cinnamon and grated nutmeg
1/4 teaspoon vanilla extract
1 tablespoon chopped pecans, toasted

Preheat broiler.

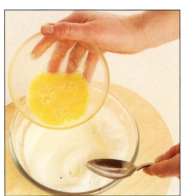

To make the filling, combine the apple, sugar, spices, and vanilla in a small saucepan. Cook over low heat, stirring occasionally, until tender. Beat the egg whites until soft peaks form. In another bowl, beat the egg until light yellow in color. Season with salt and pepper. Fold the egg into the beaten egg whites. Heat an 8-inch nonstick skillet over medium heat. Spray with cooking spray. Add the egg mixture and as the eggs set, lift to allow liquid to flow under. Cook until almost set.

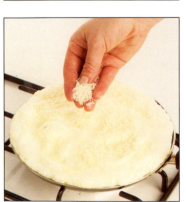

Sprinkle with Parmesan and broil until the top is set. Spoon the apple mixture on one side and fold in half. Sprinkle with the pecans.

Serves 1

Per serving: 129 Calories, Protein 15 g, Carb 1 g, Fiber 0 g, Total fat 6 g, Sat fat 2 g, Chol 216 mg, Sodium 837 mg
Exchanges: 0.9 Very Lean Meat/Protein, 1.2 Lean Meat, 0.7 Fat

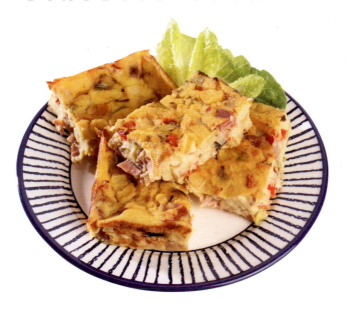

POLENTA BRUNCH BAKE

2 cups water
¹/₂ cup polenta (coarse cornmeal)
1 cup chopped leeks (white and light green parts
  only)
¹/₂ cup diced red bell pepper
2 oz prosciutto, diced
1 cup silken tofu
2 eggs
freshly ground pepper, to taste

Preheat oven to 375F (190C). Bring the water to a boil. Slowly stir in the polenta and cook, stirring, until thickened, about 10 minutes.

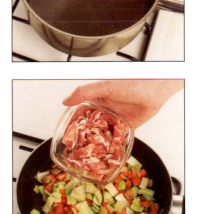

Meanwhile, spray a nonstick skillet and an 8-inch square pan with cooking spray. Add the leeks and bell pepper to the skillet and cook until softened, stirring occasionally. Add the prosciutto and cook until browned. Beat the tofu until pureed. Add the eggs, beat until light yellow, and season with pepper. Stir the egg mixture and prosciutto mixture into the polenta mixture. Transfer to the prepared pan.

Bake for 35 minutes or until the edges are brown and a knife inserted in the center comes out clean.

Serves 6

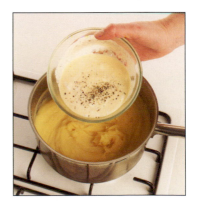

Per serving: 121 Calories, Protein 8 g, Carb 15 g, Fiber 2 g, Total fat 3 g, Sat fat 1 g, Chol 79 mg, Sodium 230 mg
Exchanges: 0.7 Bread/Starch, 1 Lean Meat, 0.6 Vegetable

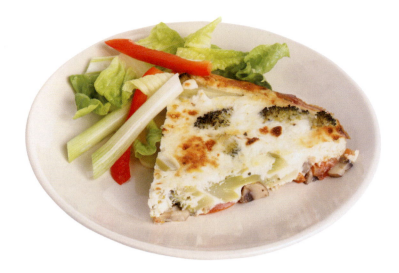

BROCCOLI FRITTATA

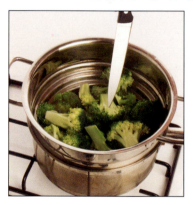

6 oz broccoli florets, cut into bite-size pieces
3 eggs
3 egg whites
freshly ground pepper, to taste
dash of hot pepper sauce
1 tablespoon olive oil
2 tablespoons finely chopped white onion
1 cup chopped fresh mushrooms
2 Roma tomatoes, chopped
1/4 cup crumbled feta cheese

Preheat broiler. Steam the broccoli over boiling water until crisp-tender, about 3 minutes.

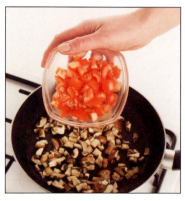

Beat the eggs, egg whites, pepper, and hot pepper sauce in a medium bowl until light. Set aside. Heat the oil in a 9-inch oven-proof skillet over medium heat. Add the onion; cook until softened. Add the mush-rooms and cook until starting to brown. Add the tomatoes. Cook for 1 minute. Arrange the broccoli evenly over the mush-room mixture and then sprinkle over the feta cheese.

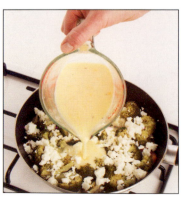

Pour over the egg mixture. Cook for 4 minutes, until the bottom is lightly browned. Broil for 2 minutes, until the top is lightly browned and the eggs are set.

Serves 6

Per serving: 96 Calories, Protein 7 g, Carb 3 g, Fiber 1 g, Total fat 6 g, Sat fat 2 g, Chol 119 mg, Sodium 137 mg
Exchanges: 0.8 Lean Meat, 0.6 Vegetable, 1 Fat

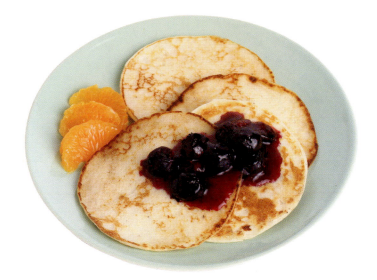

RICOTTA PANCAKES

$^1/_2$ cup all-purpose flour
$^1/_4$ cup soy flour
1 teaspoon baking powder
$^1/_4$ teaspoon salt
$^1/_8$ teaspoon freshly ground nutmeg
1 cup reduced-fat ricotta cheese
$^3/_4$ cup skim dairy milk or unsweetened soy milk
1 teaspoon vanilla extract
2 egg whites

Combine the flours, baking powder, salt, and nutmeg in a bowl.

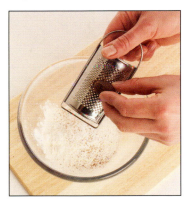

In another bowl, combine the cheese, milk, and vanilla. Stir the cheese mixture into the flour mixture until just combined. Beat the egg whites until stiff peaks form. Fold the egg whites into the batter. Drop spoonfuls onto a hot griddle or heavy bottomed pan to make 3-inch pancakes.

Cook until bubbles form. Turn and cook until the edges are dry.

Makes 16 (3-inch) pancakes; serves 4

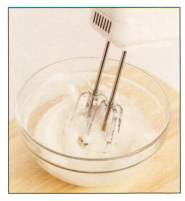

Per serving: 193 Calories, Protein 14 g, Carb 19 g, Fiber 1 g, Total fat 6 g, Sat fat 3 g, Chol 20 mg, Sodium 372 mg
Exchanges: 0.8 Bread/Starch, 1.2 Lean Meat, 0.7 Fat

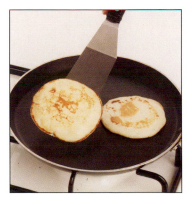

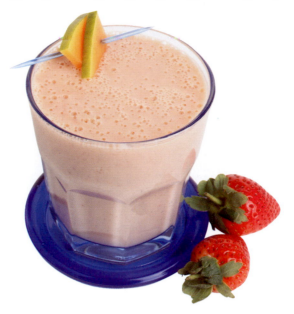

PAPAYA-STRAWBERRY SMOOTHIE

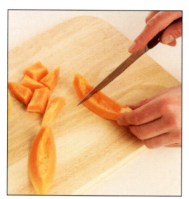

$^{1}/_{2}$ fresh papaya
1 cup strawberries
5 oz tofu (drained weight)
1 cup fresh orange or tangerine juice
$^{1}/_{2}$ cup water or as needed

Remove the seeds from the papaya and peel. Cut the flesh into cubes and add to a blender.

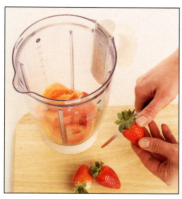

Remove the caps from the strawberries and add to the blender. Cut the tofu into 4 or 5 pieces and add to the blender with the juice.

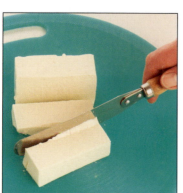

Blend until pureed. Add about $^{1}/_{2}$ cup water or enough to make a good pouring consistency. Pour into glasses and serve.

Serves 2

Per serving: 159 Calories, Protein 6 g, Carb 28 g, Fiber 4 g, Total fat 3 g, Sat fat <1 g, Chol 0 mg, Sodium 10 mg
Exchanges: 0.9 Very Lean Meat/Protein, 1.9 Fruit, 0.5 Fat

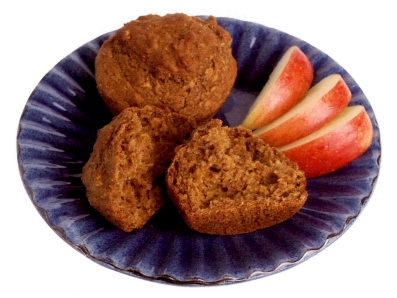

BRAN MUFFINS

2 cups high-fiber cereal
1½ cups skim milk
1 cup whole-wheat flour
½ cup soy flour
¼ cup gluten
¼ cup Splenda® Granular no calorie sweetener
1 tablespoon baking powder
1 teaspoon ground cinnamon
¼ teaspoon salt
2 tablespoons ground flaxseeds
2 tablespoons canola oil
2 eggs whites or 1 whole egg, beaten
1 tablespoon molasses
1 teaspoon vanilla extract

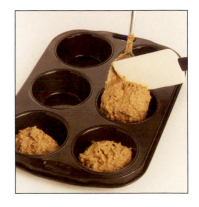

Preheat oven to 400F (200C). Spray 12 (2½–3 inch) nonstick muffin cups with cooking spray. Combine the cereal and milk in a medium bowl; let stand, stirring occasionally, for 10 minutes. In another bowl, combine the flours, gluten, Splenda®, baking powder, cinnamon, and salt. Stir the flaxseeds, oil, egg whites, molasses, and vanilla into the cereal mixture. Stir in the dry ingredients until just moistened.

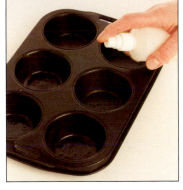

Spoon the batter into the prepared pan, mounding batter in cups. Bake for 20 minutes or until the muffins spring back when lightly pressed.

Makes 12 muffins

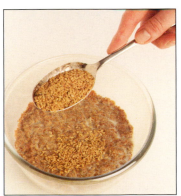

Per muffin: 136 Calories, Protein 6 g, Carb 20 g, Fiber 5 g, Total fat 4 g, Sat fat <1 g, Chol 0 mg, Sodium 196 mg
Exchanges: 1.1 Vegetable, 0.7 Fat

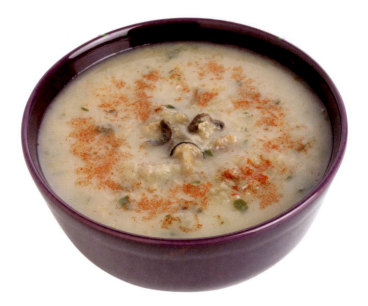

DOUBLE OYSTER BISQUE

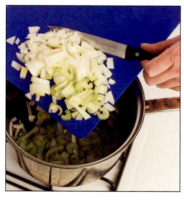

1/2 tablespoon olive oil
1/2 tablespoon no-trans fat margarine or butter
2 stalks celery, finely chopped
1/4 cup finely chopped leek (white part only)
1 tablespoon chopped fresh parsley
1 teaspoon fresh thyme or 1/2 teaspoon dried
4 oz fresh oyster mushrooms, cleaned
2 cups reduced-sodium chicken broth
2 tablespoons dry sherry
dash of Worcestershire sauce
dash of hot pepper sauce
24 fresh oysters
2 cups 2% calcium-fortified milk or fat-free half-
   and-half whisked with 1 tablespoon cornstarch
salt and white pepper, to taste
cayenne or paprika, for garnish

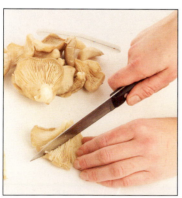

Heat the oil and margarine in a large saucepan over medium heat. Add the celery, leek, parsley, and thyme. Sauté until the vegetables are tender but not browned, stirring frequently. Discard the mushroom stems and coarsely chop. Add to the saucepan and cook, stirring occasionally, for 5 minutes. Add the broth, sherry, and sauces. Simmer until the vegetables are tender, about 5 minutes. Remove the oysters from their shells, add, and simmer until the edges curl, about 5 minutes. Transfer, in batches, to a food processor and finely chop.

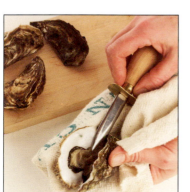

Return to a clean saucepan. Add the milk and season with salt and pepper. Over low heat, stir until hot and slightly thickened. Ladle into bowls and sprinkle with cayenne.

Makes 6 (1-cup) servings

Per cup: 156 Calories, Protein 12 g, Carb 13 g, Fiber <1 g, Total fat 6 g, Sat fat 2 g, Chol 48 mg, Sodium 198 mg
Exchanges: 1 Very Lean Meat/Protein, 1 Fat

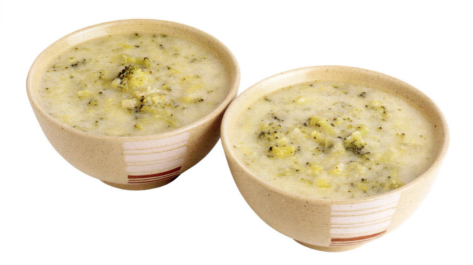

CREAMY BROCCOLI SOUP

¹/₂ tablespoon olive oil
¹/₂ tablespoon no-trans fat margarine or butter
1¹/₂ cups finely chopped leek (light green and white parts only)
4 cups reduced-sodium chicken broth
1 lb fresh or frozen broccoli florets
2 cups 1% calcium-fortified milk or fat-free half-and-half whisked with 1 tablespoon cornstarch
¹/₂ cup (2 oz) grated cheddar cheese
salt and freshly ground pepper, to taste

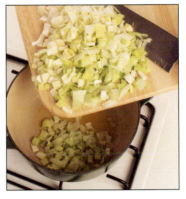

Heat the oil and margarine in a Dutch oven over medium heat. Add the leek and sauté until tender but not browned, stirring frequently.

Add the broth and bring to a boil. Add the broccoli and bring to a boil. Reduce heat to low, cover, and simmer until the broccoli is very tender and soft, about 15 minutes. Break up the broccoli with a wooden spoon or whisk. Stir in the milk and simmer, stirring, until hot and slightly thickened, about 5 minutes.

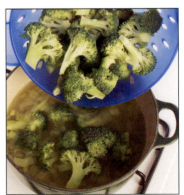

Remove from the heat and whisk in the cheese until melted. Taste and season with salt and pepper.

Makes 6 (1-cup) servings

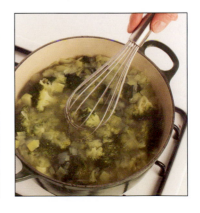

> **Per cup:** 147 Calories, Protein 10 g, Carb 13 g, Fiber 3 g, Total fat 7 g, Sat fat 4 g, Chol 18 mg, Sodium 261 mg
> **Exchanges:** 0.5 Lean Meat/Protein, 1.5 Vegetable, 1 Fat

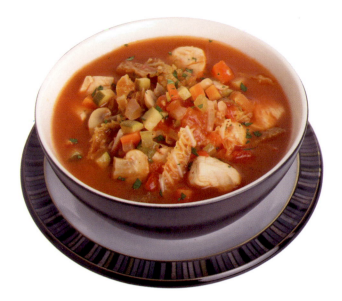

— CHICKEN & VEGETABLE SOUP —

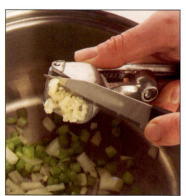

1 tablespoon olive oil
1 medium onion, chopped
2 stalks celery, chopped
1 clove garlic, minced
2 boneless, skinless chicken breast halves, cut into
  bite-size pieces
1 (14½-oz) can diced tomatoes
4 cups reduced-sodium chicken broth
2 carrots, chopped
1 zucchini, chopped
4 oz button mushrooms, sliced
1 cup shredded cabbage
salt and freshly ground black pepper, to taste
chopped fresh parsley, for garnish

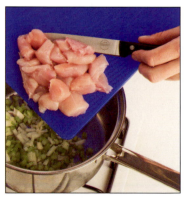

Heat the oil in a large saucepan over medium heat. Add the onion, celery, and garlic and cook until softened. Add the chicken and cook, stirring, until no longer pink. Add the tomatoes with juice, broth, and carrots. Bring to a boil. Reduce heat, cover, and simmer for 10 minutes. Add the zucchini, mushrooms, and cabbage. Cover and simmer until the vegetables and chicken are tender, about 20 minutes.

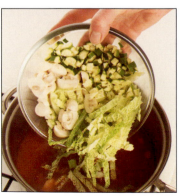

Season with salt and pepper. Ladle into bowls. Top with parsley.

Makes 7 (1-cup) servings

Per cup: 117 Calories, Protein 11 g, Carb 11 g, Fiber 3 g, Total fat 3 g, Sat fat <1 g, Chol 22 mg, Sodium 188 mg
Exchanges: 1 Very Lean Meat/Protein, 1.5 Vegetable

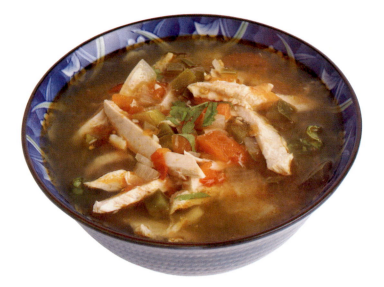

CHICKEN-LIME SOUP

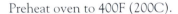

4 cups water
2 cups reduced-sodium chicken broth
2 boneless, skinless chicken breast halves
1 small onion, sliced
1 bay leaf and 1 parsley sprig
3 corn tortillas (optional)
1/2 tablespoon olive oil
1 small onion, chopped
1 clove garlic, minced
1/2 green bell pepper, finely chopped
2 medium tomatoes, finely chopped
1/2 serrano chili, seeded and minced, or to taste
salt and freshly ground pepper, to taste
juice of 1 lime, plus lime wedges to serve
fresh cilantro leaves, for garnish

Preheat oven to 400F (200C).

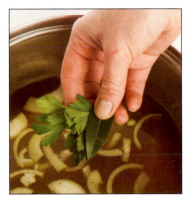

Combine the water, broth, chicken, onion, bay leaf, and parsley in a saucepan. Simmer for 20 minutes until the chicken is very tender. Strain the broth into a bowl. Shred the chicken. If using, stack the tortillas and cut into matchstick-size pieces. Arrange on a baking sheet. Spray with cooking spray and toss. Bake for 5 minutes, until crisp. Heat the oil in a saucepan. Add the onion, garlic, bell pepper, tomatoes, and chili. Cook until softened, stirring occasionally. Add the broth and chicken. Simmer until the vegetables are tender, 5–10 minutes.

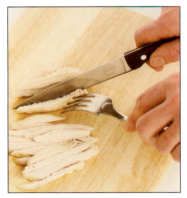

Season with salt and pepper. Stir in the lime juice and ladle into bowls. Top with tortillas and cilantro. Serve with lime wedges.

Makes 6 (1-cup) servings

Per cup: 93 Calories, Protein 11 g, Carb 7 g, Fiber 2 g, Total fat 2 g, Sat fat <1 g, Chol 24 mg, Sodium 66 mg
Exchanges: 1 Very Lean Meat/Protein, 1 Vegetable

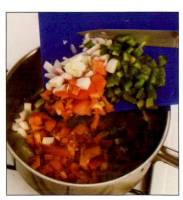

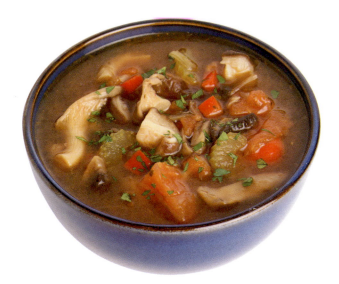

MIXED MUSHROOM SOUP

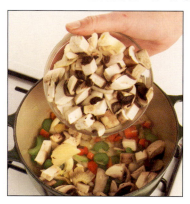

2 tablespoons olive oil
$1/2$ cup chopped white onion
$1/2$ cup chopped red bell pepper
$1/4$ cup finely chopped celery
1 lb mixed mushrooms, chopped
4 cups chicken broth
8 oz fresh tomatoes, chopped
1 bay leaf
$1/2$ teaspoon dried oregano
2 tablespoons dry sherry
salt and freshly ground pepper, to taste
dash of hot pepper sauce
1 tablespoon fresh parsley, finely chopped

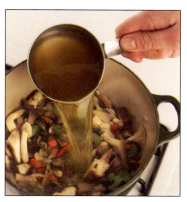

Heat the oil in a Dutch oven over medium heat. Add the onion, bell pepper, and celery and cook for 5 minutes. Add the mushrooms and cook for about 5 minutes, until the mushrooms are softened and begin to release their juice. Add the broth, tomatoes, bay leaf, oregano, and sherry. Simmer over low heat for 20 minutes or until the vegetables are tender, the flavors are blended, and the soup is slightly reduced.

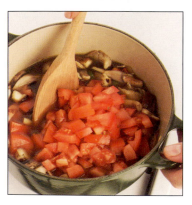

Season with salt, pepper, and hot pepper sauce. Discard the bay leaf. Stir in the parsley and serve.

Makes 4 (1$1/2$-cup) servings

Per cup: 103 Calories, Protein 5 g, Carb 8 g, Fiber 2 g, Total fat 6 g, Sat fat 1 g, Chol 3 mg, Sodium 84 mg
Exchanges: 1.5 Vegetable, 1 Fat

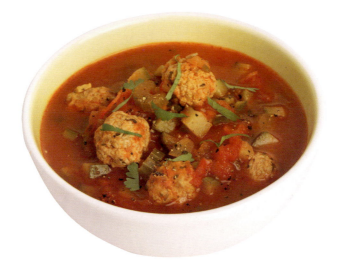

MEXICAN MEATBALL SOUP

1 tablespoon olive oil
1 medium white onion, chopped
1 stalk celery, finely chopped
4 cups reduced-sodium chicken broth
1 cup water
1 (14½-oz) can diced tomatoes
1 bay leaf
1 parsley sprig
1 (4-oz) can diced mild green chilies
2 small zucchini, chopped
8 oz lean ground turkey
1 clove garlic, minced
¼ teaspoon dried thyme
¼ teaspoon salt
freshly ground black pepper, to taste
fresh cilantro leaves, to serve

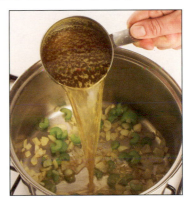

Heat the oil in a large saucepan over medium heat. Add the onion and celery and cook until softened. Add the broth, water, tomatoes with juice, bay leaf, parsley sprig, chilies, and zucchini. Bring to a boil. Reduce the heat, cover, and simmer over low heat until the vegetables are tender, about 15 minutes. Meanwhile, combine the turkey, garlic, thyme, salt, and pepper in a small bowl. Using a slightly heaped measuring teaspoon, shape into about 28 balls. Add the meatballs to the saucepan.

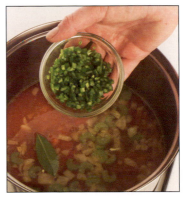

Simmer until the meatballs rise to the surface and are cooked through, about 5 minutes. Discard the bay leaf and parsley. Ladle into bowls and top with cilantro.

Makes 8 (1-cup) servings

Per cup: 106 Calories, Protein 8 g, Carb 7 g, Fiber 2 g, Total fat 5 g, Sat fat 1 g, Chol 24 mg, Sodium 265 mg
Exchanges: 1 Lean Meat/Protein, 1 Vegetable

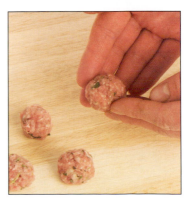

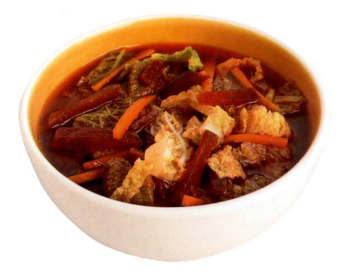

HOT BEEF BORSCHT

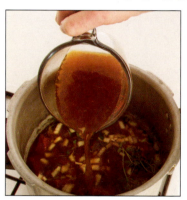

1 lb lean beef, cut into 1-inch cubes
1¼ cups chopped white onions
1 clove garlic, minced
1 bay leaf
1 parsley sprig
1 thyme sprig
4 cups reduced-sodium beef broth
3–4 cups water
1 cup shredded carrot
3 cups shredded cabbage
1 (15-oz) can shredded beets, drained, or 2 cups
  shredded fresh beets
2 tablespoons wine vinegar
2 teaspoons brown sugar
salt and freshly ground black pepper, to taste
plain low-fat yogurt, to serve (optional)

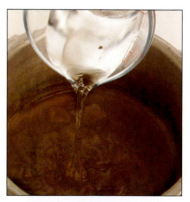

Combine the beef, onions, garlic, bay leaf, parsley, thyme, and broth in a pressure cooker. Cook at High pressure for about 10 minutes or until the beef is tender. (Or simmer in a Dutch oven over a medium-high heat for about 1 hour.) Discard the herbs. Add the water, carrot, cabbage, beets, vinegar, and brown sugar. Cook at High pressure for 10 minutes or until the vegetables are tender. (Or simmer until the vegetables are tender, about 25 minutes.) Serve with dollops of yogurt (if using).

Makes 8 (1-cup) servings

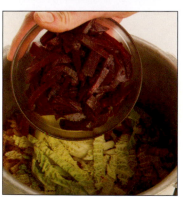

Note: leftover roast beef can be substituted for the beef.

Per cup: 180 Calories, Protein 21 g, Carb 11 g, Fiber 2 g, Total fat 6 g, Sat fat 2 g, Chol 49 mg, Sodium 189 mg
Exchanges: 3 Very Lean Meat/Protein, 1.5 Vegetable, 1 Fat

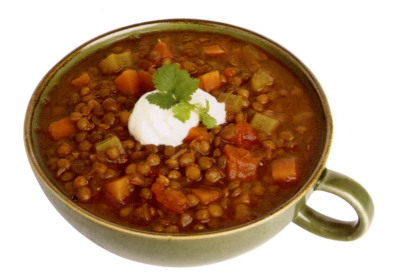

CURRIED LENTIL SOUP

1 tablespoon olive oil
1 medium white onion, chopped
2 large celery stalks, chopped
1 large carrot, chopped
2 teaspoons ground coriander
1 teaspoon ground cumin
1 teaspoon sweet paprika
$1/4$ teaspoon ground cinnamon
$1/4$ teaspoon ground turmeric
pinch of ground cloves
1 (1-lb) package green lentils, picked over and rinsed
8 cups reduced-sodium chicken broth
4 cups water, or as needed
1 ($14^1/_2$-oz) can diced tomatoes
salt and freshly ground pepper, to taste
plain nonfat yogurt and fresh cilantro leaves, for garnish

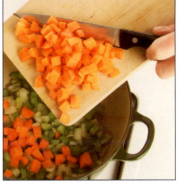

Heat the oil in a Dutch oven over medium heat. Add the onion and celery and sauté until softened. Add the carrot and spices and stir to combine. Add the lentils, broth, and water. Cover and simmer until lentils are tender, about 45 minutes, adding water if needed and stirring occasionally. Stir in the tomatoes with juice. Simmer for 10 minutes to allow the flavors to blend. Season with salt and pepper. Ladle into serving bowls. Top with a dollop of yogurt and cilantro.

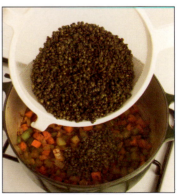

Makes 10 (1-cup) servings

Note: if desired, 4 teaspoons of good-quality curry powder can be substituted for the spices.

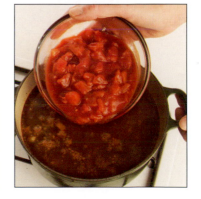

Per cup: 216 Calories, Protein 14 g, Carb 34 g, Fiber 9 g, Total fat 3 g, Sat fat <1 g, Chol 3 mg, Sodium 168 mg
Exchanges: 2 Bread/Starch, 0.5 Lean Meat/Protein, 1 Vegetable

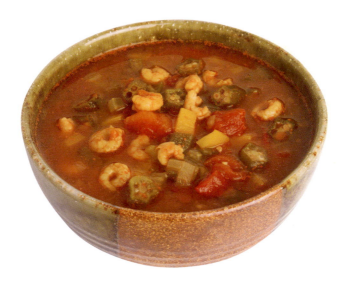

SHRIMP GUMBO

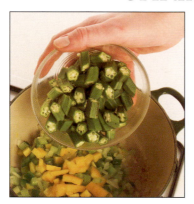

1 tablespoon olive oil
1 medium white onion, chopped
2 cloves garlic, minced
2 stalks celery, chopped
1 green bell pepper, chopped
12 oz fresh okra, trimmed and sliced, or 2$^{1}/_{2}$ cups
   frozen sliced okra
3 cups reduced-sodium chicken broth
3 cups water
$^{1}/_{2}$ cup dry white wine
1 (14$^{1}/_{2}$-oz) can diced tomatoes
1 teaspoon fresh thyme or $^{1}/_{2}$ teaspoon dried
1 lb small cooked shrimp, deveined and peeled
hot pepper sauce or cayenne, to taste
salt and freshly ground black pepper, to taste
cooked brown rice, for serving (optional)

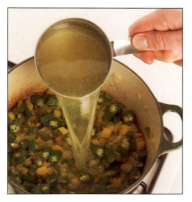

Heat the oil in a Dutch oven over medium heat. Add the onion, garlic, and celery and sauté until softened. Stir in the bell pepper and okra. Cook, stirring, until the okra begins to brown and loses its stringiness. Add the broth, water, wine, tomatoes with juice, and thyme. Bring to a boil. Reduce heat, cover, and simmer until vegetables are tender.

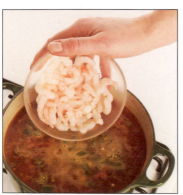

Add the shrimp. Season with hot pepper sauce, salt, and pepper. Serve over rice (if liked).

Makes 9 (1-cup) servings

Per cup: 123 Calories, Protein 13 g, Carb 10 g, Fiber 3 g, Total fat 3 g, Sat fat <1 g, Chol 78 mg, Sodium 182 mg
Exchanges: 1.5 Very Lean Meat/Protein, 1.5 Vegetable, 0.5 Fat

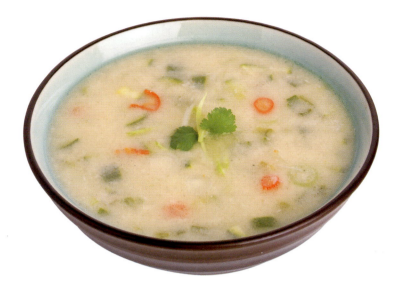

THAI CRAB SOUP

1 (14-oz) can light coconut milk
1/4 cup chopped green onions (white part only)
1 clove garlic, minced
1/2-inch piece peeled fresh ginger, julienned
1 small green bell pepper, diced
2 small zucchini, diced
1 stalk lemon grass (bottom 4–5 inches), crushed
1 hot red chili, seeded and minced
2 1/2 cups reduced-sodium chicken broth
4–6 oz fresh or frozen crabmeat, picked over for
   shell and cartilage
fresh cilantro leaves and sliced green onion tops,
   for garnish

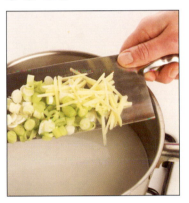

Heat 1/4 cup of the coconut milk in a large saucepan over medium-high heat. Add the onions, garlic, and ginger and cook, stirring occasionally, until softened. Add the bell pepper, zucchini, lemon grass, chili, remaining coconut milk, and broth. Bring to a boil. Reduce heat, cover, and simmer until the vegetables are tender.

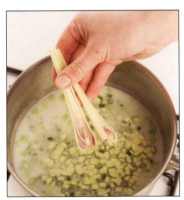

Add the crabmeat and simmer until hot. Discard the lemon grass. Ladle into bowls. Garnish with cilantro and green onion tops.

Makes 4 (1-cup) servings

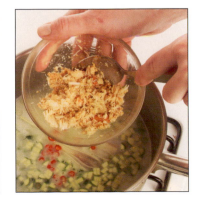

Per cup: 128 Calories, Protein 8 g, Carb 4 g,
Fiber < 1 g, Total fat 8 g, Sat fat 7 g, Chol 28 mg,
Sodium 164 mg
Exchanges: 1 Very Lean Meat/Protein

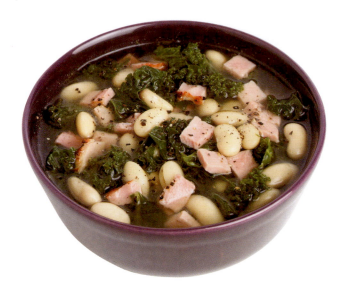

BEAN, KALE, & HAM SOUP

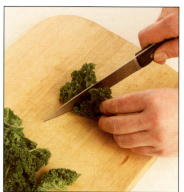

1 (10-oz) bunch fresh kale
4 cups reduced-sodium chicken broth
4 cups water
2 (15-oz) cans no-salt added white beans (navy,
   Great Northern, or cannellini), drained and rinsed,
   or 3 cups cooked beans
1 cup chopped cooked ham
freshly ground pepper, to taste
dash of hot pepper sauce

Rinse and dry the kale. Discard large stems
and cut the leaves into bite-size pieces.

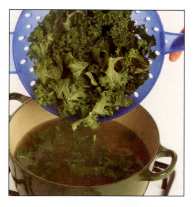

Bring the broth and water to a boil in a
Dutch oven. Add the kale and cook until
bright green and wilted. Reduce heat, cover,
and simmer for about 15 minutes or until
the kale is tender.

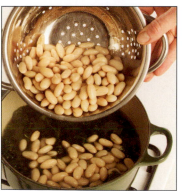

Add the beans and ham. Simmer for 10
minutes to blend the flavors. Season with
pepper and hot pepper sauce.

Makes 8 (1-cup) servings

Per cup: 206 Calories, Protein 15 g, Carb 34 g,
Fiber 7 g, Total fat 2 g, Sat fat 1 g, Chol 10 mg,
Sodium 311 mg
Exchanges: 2 Bread/Starch, 1.4 Lean
Meat/Protein, 1 Vegetable

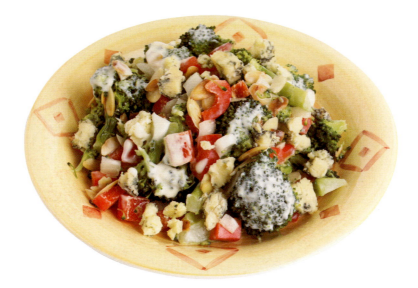

BROCCOLI SALAD

8 oz (4 cups) bite-size broccoli florets
2 tablespoons fat-free sour cream or yogurt
2 tablespoons reduced-fat mayonnaise
1/2 teaspoon Dijon mustard
1/4 teaspoon sugar
1 red bell pepper, roasted, peeled, and chopped (see
   page 72)
1/4 cup diced white onion
2–4 tablespoons slivered almonds
2–4 tablespoons crumbled blue cheese
salt and freshly ground pepper, to taste

Steam the broccoli florets for 3 minutes
until bright green and crisp-tender.

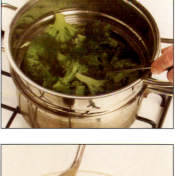

Combine the sour cream, mayonnaise,
mustard, and sugar in a small bowl.
Combine the broccoli, bell pepper, onion,
almonds, and cheese in a large bowl. Add
the dressing and toss to combine. Season
with salt and pepper. Cover and refrigerate
for about 1 hour before serving to allow the
flavors to blend.

Makes about 8 side-salad servings

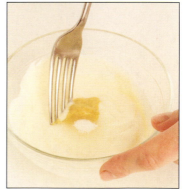

Note: this salad can be stored, covered, in
the refrigerator for 2–3 days.

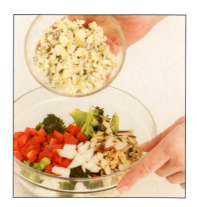

Per serving: 58 Calories, Protein 2 g, Carb 5 g,
Fiber 2 g, Total fat 3 g, Sat fat <1 g, Chol 3 mg,
Sodium 158 mg
Exchanges: 0.5 Fruit, 0.5 Vegetable, 0.5 Fat

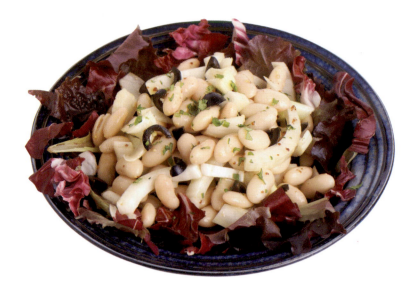

— WHITE BEAN-FENNEL SALAD —

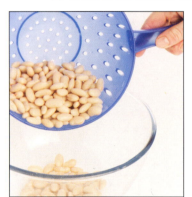

1 (15-oz) can cannellini (white kidney beans)
1 small fennel bulb with leaves
2 tablespoons extra-virgin olive oil
1 tablespoon sherry vinegar
1 teaspoon whole grain mustard
1 tablespoon diced Kalamata olives
freshly ground pepper, to taste
radicchio leaves, to serve

Drain the beans, rinse with cold water, and drain again. Transfer to a medium bowl.

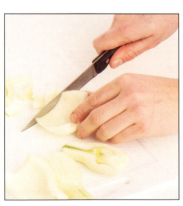

Separate the fennel, rinse, and cut crosswise into $1/4$-inch wide pieces about 2 inches long. Mince 1 tablespoon of the leaves and reserve some whole fronds for garnish. Whisk the oil, vinegar, and mustard in a small bowl. Pour over the beans and toss to combine. Stir in the olives and 1 tablespoon fennel leaves and season with pepper.

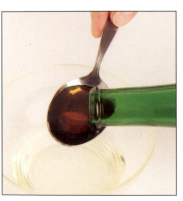

Cover and refrigerate for 1 hour to allow the flavors to blend. Spoon into the radicchio leaves. Garnish with reserved fennel fronds.

Makes 4 side salads or 2 main-dish salads

Per side serving: 175 Calories, Protein 5 g, Carb 19 g, Fiber 6 g, Total fat 9 g, Sat fat 1 g, Chol 0 mg, Sodium 344 mg
Exchanges: 1 Bread/Starch, 1 Vegetable, 1.5 Fat

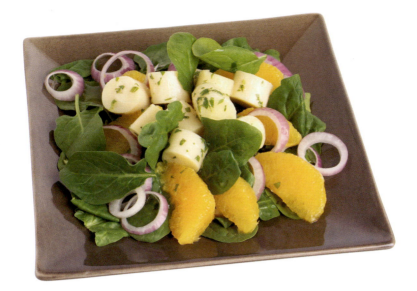

HEARTS OF PALM SALAD

1 (14-oz) can hearts of palm
¹/₄ cup fresh tangerine or orange juice
2 tablespoons olive oil
1 teaspoon minced fresh mint or ¹/₂ teaspoon dried
dash of salt (optional)
6 cups baby spinach leaves, rinsed and dried
2 oranges
1 small red onion, separated into rings

Drain the hearts of palm and rinse. Cut the stalks crosswise into ¹/₂-inch pieces; set aside.

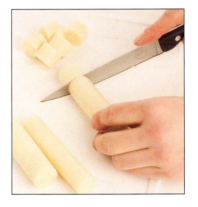

Combine the juice, oil, mint, and salt (if using) in a small bowl. Whisk to combine and pour over the hearts of palm. Toss gently to combine. Divide the spinach among 4 salad plates.

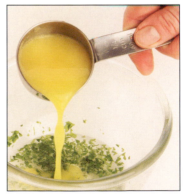

Peel and segment the oranges, then add to the salad with the onion rings. Spoon the hearts of palm and dressing over the salads and serve.

Makes 4 side salad servings

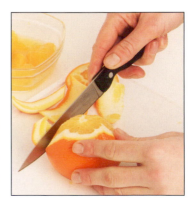

Per serving: 148 Calories, Protein 5 g, Carb 18 g, Fiber 6 g, Total fat 8 g, Sat fat 1 g, Chol 0 mg, Sodium 533 mg
Exchanges: 1 Fruit, 1 Vegetable, 1 Fat

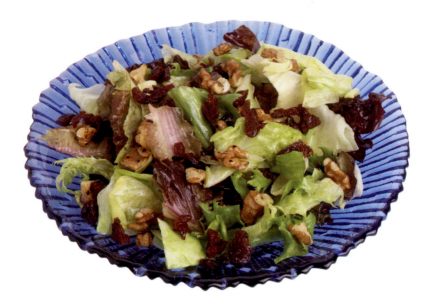

— WALNUT-CHERRY GREENS —

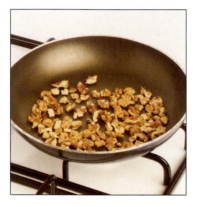

¹/4 cup walnuts, broken into coarse pieces
1 tablespoon extra-virgin olive oil
1 tablespoon walnut oil
2 tablespoons fresh lemon juice
2 tablespoons water or reduced-fat chicken broth
2 teaspoons Dijon mustard
pinch of sugar
6 cups mixed salad greens, rinsed and dried
¹/4 cup dried sweet cherries, coarsely chopped

Toast the walnuts in a dry skillet over medium heat, until fragrant and beginning to brown, stirring occasionally. Set aside.

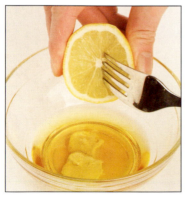

Combine the oils, lemon juice, water, mustard, and sugar in a small bowl. Whisk to combine and dissolve sugar.

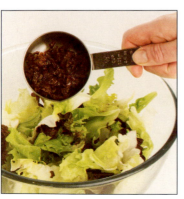

Combine the greens, walnuts, and cherries in a large bowl. Add the dressing and toss to coat. Serve immediately.

Serves 4

Per serving: 158 Calories, Protein 3 g, Carb 10 g, Fiber 3 g, Total fat 12 g, Sat fat 1 g, Chol 0 mg, Sodium 90 mg
Exchanges: 0.5 Fruit, 0.5 Vegetable, 2 Fat

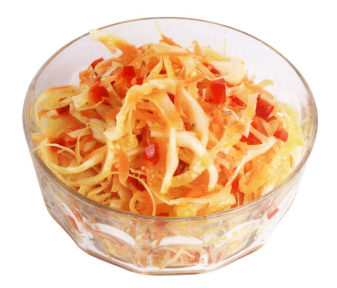

COLESLAW WITH VINAIGRETTE

3 cups finely shredded cabbage
1 large carrot, shredded
1 small red bell pepper, diced
3 tablespoons canola oil
2 tablespoons white wine vinegar
1 packet Splenda® no calorie sweetener or 1
   teaspoon sugar
1 teaspoon celery seeds (optional)
salt and freshly ground pepper, to taste

Combine the cabbage, carrot, and bell pepper in a large bowl.

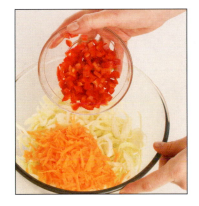

Add the oil, vinegar, Splenda®, celery seeds (if using), salt, and pepper to a small bowl. Whisk until combined.

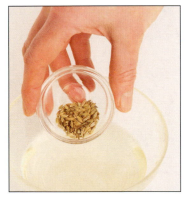

Add the dressing to the cabbage mixture and toss to combine. The coleslaw can be refrigerated for up to 2 days.

Serves 4–6

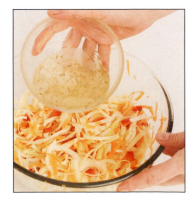

Per serving: 125 Calories, Protein 1 g, Carb 7 g,
Fiber 2 g, Total fat 11 g, Sat fat <1 g, Chol 0 mg,
Sodium 24 mg
Exchanges: 1.5 Vegetable, 2 Fat

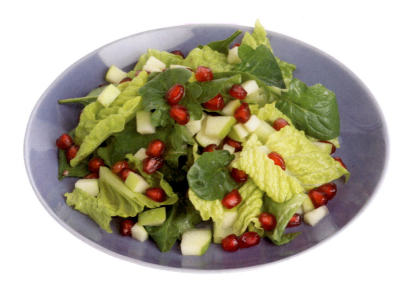

APPLE-SPINACH SALAD

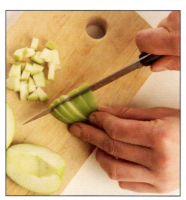

1 Granny Smith apple
2 tablespoons fresh lemon juice
1 pomegranate
4 cups baby spinach leaves
2 cups bite-size pieces romaine lettuce
2 tablespoons extra-virgin olive oil
2 tablespoons unsweetened apple juice
1 teaspoon Dijon mustard

Cut the apple into quarters and core. Finely chop apple and add to a large bowl. Stir in 1 teaspoon of the lemon juice and toss to combine.

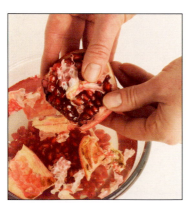

To separate the pomegranate seeds, score the skin lengthwise in several places and cut off ends. Holding the fruit under water, break apart into sections. Separate the seeds from the membranes; the seeds will sink and membranes and other bits will float. Discard membranes and any floating bits. Drain seeds and pat dry with paper towels. Use half the seeds for the salad and refrigerate the remaining seeds for another use. Add the spinach and romaine to the apple.

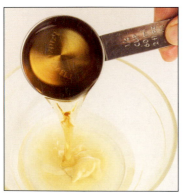

Add the remaining lemon juice, oil, apple juice, and mustard to a small bowl and whisk. Add to the spinach and toss. Sprinkle with the pomegranate seeds.

Serves 4

Per serving: 110 Calories, Protein 2 g, Carb 11 g, Fiber 2 g, Total fat 7 g, Sat fat 1 g, Chol 0 mg, Sodium 107 mg
Exchanges: 0.5 Fruit, 0.5 Vegetable, 1 Fat

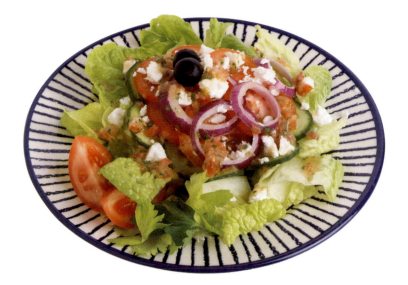

CUCUMBER & TOMATO SALAD

$^1/_2$ greenhouse cucumber
3 Roma tomatoes
1 small red onion
$^1/_4$ cup crumbled feta cheese
lettuce leaves, to serve
Kalamata olives, for garnish (optional)
HERB-TOMATO DRESSING:
$^1/_3$ cup chopped fresh tomato
1 tablespoon white wine vinegar
1 tablespoon extra-virgin olive oil
1 clove garlic, minced
1 tablespoon chopped fresh parsley
2 teaspoons chopped fresh basil or 1 teaspoon dried
1 teaspoon chopped fresh oregano or $^1/_2$ teaspoon dried
salt and freshly ground pepper, to taste

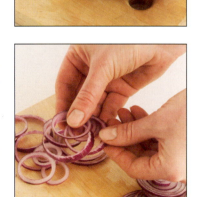

Thinly slice the cucumber crosswise. Transfer to a shallow glass dish. Slice the tomatoes crosswise. Peel the onion, cut into thin crosswise slices, and separate into rings. Top the cucumber with the tomatoes, onion, and feta. Add the dressing ingredients to a mini food processor or blender. Process until combined. Add water if needed to make a thin pouring consistency. Pour dressing over salad. Cover and refrigerate for 1 hour.

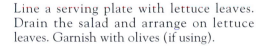

Line a serving plate with lettuce leaves. Drain the salad and arrange on lettuce leaves. Garnish with olives (if using).

Serves 6

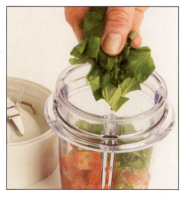

Per serving: 58 Calories, Protein 2 g, Carb 5 g, Fiber 1 g, Total fat 4 g, Sat fat 1 g, Chol 5 mg, Sodium 74 mg
Exchanges: 1 Vegetable, 1 Fat

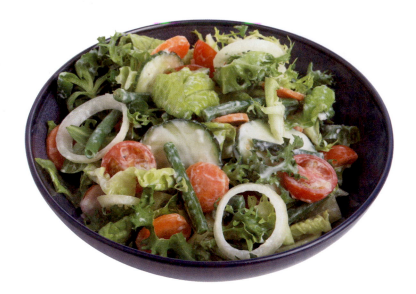

THROUGH-THE-GARDEN SALAD

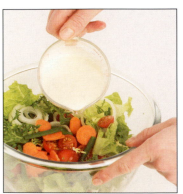

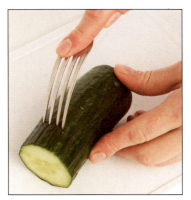

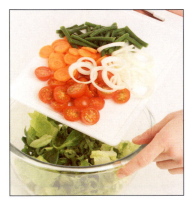

¹/₄ greenhouse cucumber
1 cup cherry tomatoes
6 cups mixed salad greens, rinsed and dried
1 medium carrot, cut into thin slices
3–4 slices sweet onion, such as Vidalia, separated
   into rings
1 cup 1-inch pieces green beans, cooked until crisp-
   tender
BUTTERMILK DRESSING:
¹/₂ cup buttermilk
¹/₄ cup reduced-fat mayonnaise
1 tablespoon grated onion
1 clove garlic, minced
1 teaspoon Dijon mustard
dash of Worcestershire sauce
salt and freshly ground pepper, to taste

Add all the dressing ingredients to a bowl
and whisk until combined. Score the skin of
the cucumber with a fork and cut crosswise
into thin slices. If the cherry tomatoes are
large, cut them into halves or quarters

Add the greens, cucumber, tomatoes, carrot,
onion, and green beans to a large bowl. Add
enough of the dressing to just coat and toss
to combine.

Serves 6

Per serving: 60 Calories, Protein 3 g, Carb 11 g,
Fiber 3 g, Total fat 1 g, Sat fat 0 g, Chol 0 mg,
Sodium 164 mg
Exchanges: 1.5 Vegetable

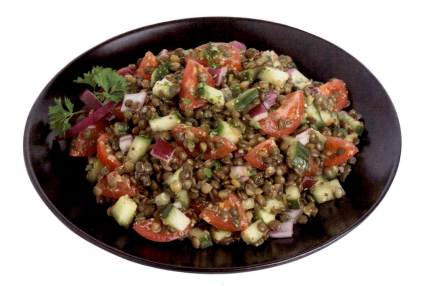

LENTIL-VEGETABLE SALAD

1 cup Le Puy green lentils
4 cups water
2 tablespoons extra-virgin olive oil
2 tablespoons seasoned rice vinegar
1 tablespoon coarse-grain mustard
1/2 teaspoon cumin seeds or 1/4 teaspoon ground
pinch of sugar
1/2 cup chopped red onion
1/2–1 cup chopped cucumber
1 cup currant tomatoes, halved, or chopped Roma
   tomatoes
2 tablespoons chopped fresh parsley
2 tablespoons chopped fresh cilantro

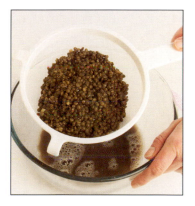

Add the lentils and water to a large saucepan and bring to a boil. Boil for 5 minutes. Reduce heat, cover, and simmer for about 20 minutes or until the lentils are just tender, stirring occasionally and adding water if needed. Drain the lentils and set aside. Grind the cumin seeds, if necessary. Add the oil, vinegar, mustard, cumin, and sugar to a small bowl. Whisk to combine. Pour over the warm lentils and gently toss to coat. Cool to room temperature.

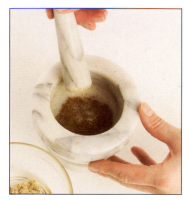

Add the remaining ingredients and gently toss to combine. Serve at room temperature or chill before serving.

Serves 6

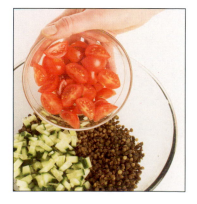

Per serving: 157 Calories, Protein 8 g, Carb 21 g,
Fiber 5 g, Total fat 5 g, Sat fat <1 g, Chol 0 mg,
Sodium 57 mg
Exchanges: 1 Bread/Starch, 0.5 Vegetable, 1 Fat

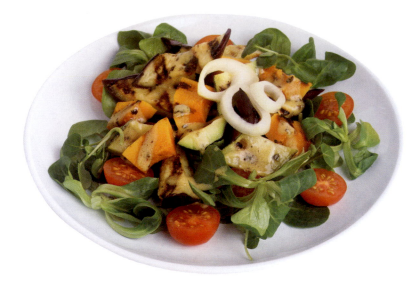

— GRILLED VEGETABLE SALAD —

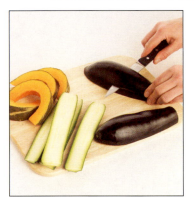

1 medium yellow summer squash
1 medium zucchini
1 Japanese eggplant (or any long slender eggplant)
4 thick slices sweet onion
2 tablespoons extra-virgin olive oil
2 tablespoons balsamic vinegar
2 teaspoons Dijon mustard
1 teaspoon dried oregano
1 teaspoon dried basil
pinch of sugar
1 cup currant or cherry tomatoes
watercress, to serve

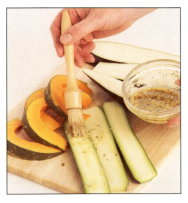

Cut the summer squash, zucchini, and egg-plant lengthwise into 3 or 4 slices depend-ing on the thickness. Add the oil, vinegar, mustard, herbs, and sugar to a small bowl. Whisk to combine. Brush the vegetables with a little of the dressing. Preheat grill or broiler. Grill the vegetables for 10–20 minutes, depending on thickness, and removing as they become crisp-tender. Cut into bite-size pieces. Transfer to a bowl and add the cherry tomatoes. Add the remaining dressing and toss to combine.

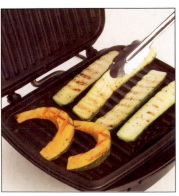

Arrange some watercress on each serving plate and top with the vegetables.

Serves 6

Per serving: 82 Calories, Protein 2 g, Carb 8 g, Fiber 2 g, Total fat 5 g, Sat fat 1 g, Chol 0 mg, Sodium 53 mg
Exchanges: 1 Vegetable, 1 Fat

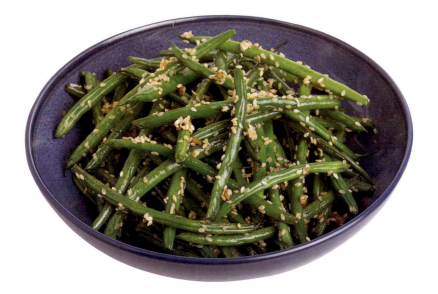

STIR-FRIED GREEN BEANS

12 oz fresh slender green beans
2 teaspoons canola oil
2 cloves garlic, minced
1 tablespoon toasted sesame seeds
salt and freshly ground pepper, to taste

Remove the ends and any strings from the green beans. Steam the beans over boiling water until almost crisp-tender.

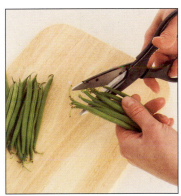

Heat the oil in a large nonstick skillet or wok. Add the garlic and cook until aromatic.

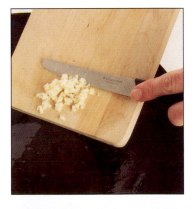

Add the beans and stir-fry until crisp-tender, about 3 minutes. Add the sesame seeds and toss to combine. Season with salt and pepper.

Serves 4

Per serving: 68 Calories, Protein 2 g, Carb 6 g, Fiber 4 g, Total fat 4 g, Sat fat <1 g, Chol 0 mg, Sodium 0 mg
Exchanges: 1 Vegetable, 0.7 Fat

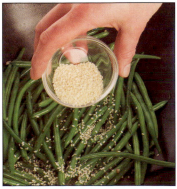

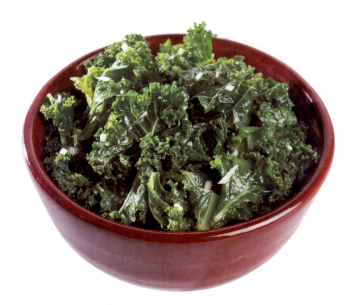

GREENS WITH GARLIC

10 oz fresh kale or collard greens
1 teaspoon olive oil
1 clove garlic, minced
1/2 cup water
salt and freshly ground black pepper, to taste

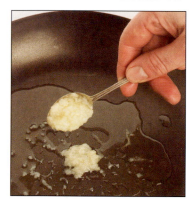

Rinse the greens to remove any sand and dirt and pat dry. Remove large stems. Place the greens on a cutting board and cut crosswise into about 1-inch pieces. Add the oil to a large skillet over medium heat. Add the garlic and cook until aromatic.

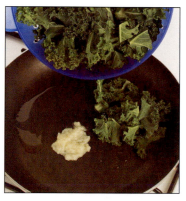

Add the greens, in batches. Then add the water and bring to a boil until kale becomes bright green.

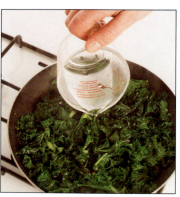

Reduce heat, cover, and simmer until tender, about 15 minutes, stirring occasionally and adding more water if needed. Drain and season with salt and pepper before serving.

Serves 4

Per serving: 47 Calories, Protein 2 g, Carb 7 g, Fiber 1 g, Total fat 2 g, Sat fat <1 g, Chol 0 mg, Sodium 30 mg
Exchanges: 1.4 Vegetable, 0.7 Fat

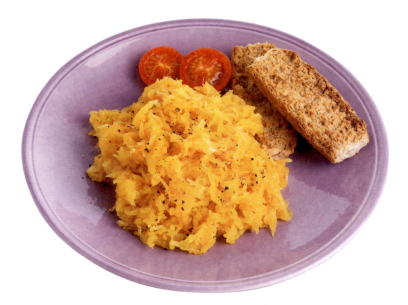

SPAGHETTI SQUASH & CHEESE

1 (about 3-lb) spaghetti squash
4 teaspoons no-trans fat margarine or butter
4 teaspoons olive oil
1/4 cup freshly grated Parmesan cheese
salt and freshly ground pepper, to taste

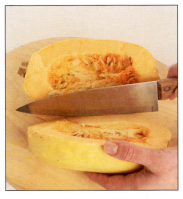

Preheat oven to 350F (180C). Spray a non-stick baking pan with cooking spray. Cut the squash in half lengthwise. Use a spoon to scrape out the seeds. Place the squash, cut sides down, in the prepared pan. Bake for 45 minutes or until the flesh is tender when probed with a fork.

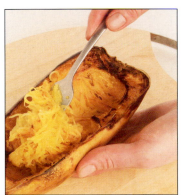

Allow the squash to cool. Using a fork, to remove the flesh in spaghetti-like strands; measure 4 cups of squash and refrigerate or freeze the remaining squash for another use. Heat the margarine and oil in a large skillet over medium heat.

Add the 4 cups of the squash and toss to heat. Add the cheese and toss to combine. Season with salt and pepper.

Serves 8

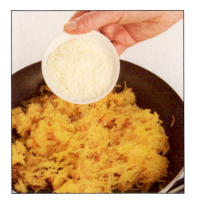

Per serving: 86 Calories, Protein 2 g, Carb 9 g,
Fiber 2 g, Total fat 5 g, Sat fat 2 g, Chol 7 mg,
Sodium 416 mg
Exchanges: 0.6 Bread/Starch, 0.9 Fat

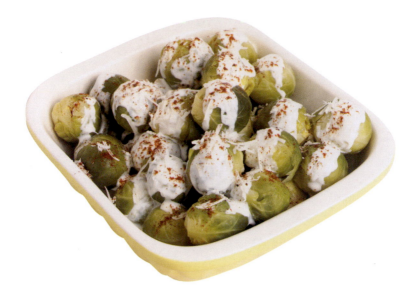

— CREAMY BRUSSELS SPROUTS —

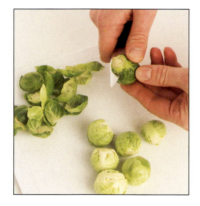

1 lb fresh Brussels sprouts, trimmed and cut in half
2 oz reduced-fat cream cheese, cut into cubes
1/3 cup skim milk
grated peel of 1 lemon
1 tablespoon freshly grated Parmesan cheese
  (optional)
sweet paprika, for garnish

Trim the root ends and remove any browned leaves from the Brussels sprouts. Cut an "X" in the ends of the stems. Cook in salted boiling water until tender, about 10 minutes.

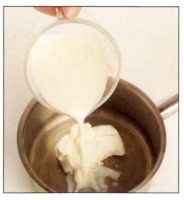

Combine the cream cheese, milk, and lemon peel in a small saucepan. Heat over low heat until cheese melts, stirring frequently.

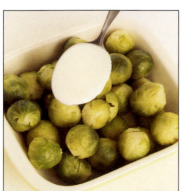

Drain the Brussels sprouts and transfer to a serving dish. Spoon the sauce over and sprinkle with the Parmesan cheese (if using) and paprika.

Serves 4

Per serving: 95 Calories, Protein 6 g, Carb 12 g, Fiber 4 g, Total fat 3 g, Sat fat 2 g, Chol 9 mg, Sodium 104 mg
Exchanges: 1.9 Vegetable

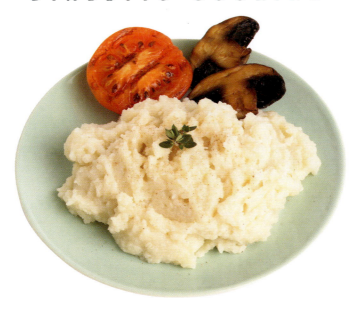

WHIPPED CAULIFLOWER

1 medium head cauliflower
1 tablespoon freshly grated Parmesan cheese
1 tablespoon no-trans fat margarine or butter
1/2 cup reduced-sodium chicken broth or skim milk
salt and white pepper, to taste
freshly grated nutmeg, to taste

Discard the green leaves and cut the cauliflower into florets.

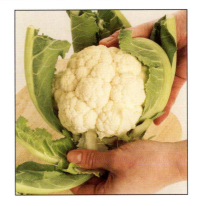

Cook the cauliflower in a large pan of salted boiling water until very tender, about 10 minutes. Drain and transfer to a food processor. Pulse until pureed.

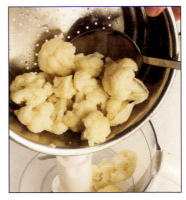

Add the cheese, margarine, and enough broth to make the consistency of mashed potatoes, pulsing to combine. Season with salt, pepper, and nutmeg.

Serves 4

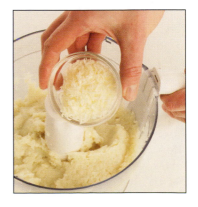

Per serving: 71 Calories, Protein 4 g, Carb 8 g, Fiber 4 g, Total fat 4 g, Sat fat 1 g, Chol 9 mg, Sodium 109 mg
Exchanges: 1.4 Vegetable, 0.6 Fat

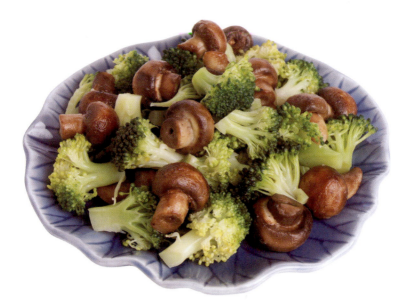

BROCCOLI WITH MUSHROOMS

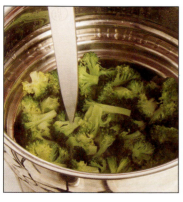

6 oz fresh crimini (baby portobello) mushrooms
12 oz small broccoli florets or fresh broccolini (baby broccoli)
1 tablespoon no-trans fat margarine or butter
salt and freshly ground black pepper, to taste

Wipe the mushrooms clean with a damp paper towel or brush lightly to remove dirt. Leave whole, or cut into quarters if large, and set aside.

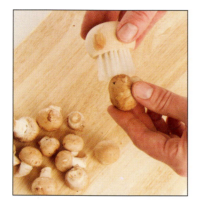

Steam the broccoli over boiling water until tender, about 8 minutes. Transfer to a serving dish. Melt the margarine in a skillet over medium-high heat. Add the mushrooms and sauté until starting to brown, stirring frequently.

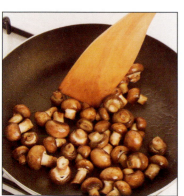

Add the mushrooms to the broccoli, mix together, and serve.

Serves 4

Per serving: 71 Calories, Protein 4 g, Carb 8 g, Fiber 2 g, Total fat 3 g, Sat fat 1 g, Chol 0 mg, Sodium 59 mg
Exchanges: 1.6 Vegetable, 0.6 Fat

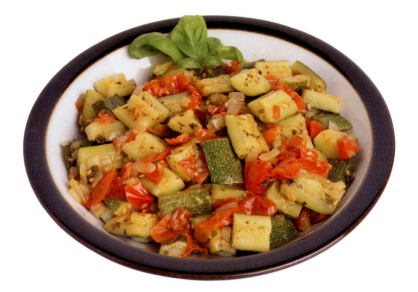

ZUCCHINI & TOMATOES

2 (8-oz) zucchini
1/2 cup chopped onion
1 teaspoon fresh chopped oregano or 1/2 teaspoon dried
1 teaspoon fresh chopped basil or 1/2 teaspoon dried
1 cup water
4 Roma tomatoes, chopped
salt and freshly ground pepper, to taste

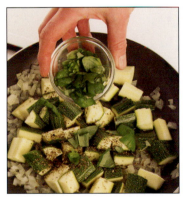

Cut the ends off the zucchini and cut into quarters. Slice crosswise into 1/2-inch slices.

Spray a nonstick skillet with cooking spray. Add the onion and cook over medium heat, stirring occasionally, until softened. Add the zucchini, herbs, and water. Bring to a boil. Reduce heat, cover, and simmer until the zucchini is crisp-tender, about 15 minutes, stirring occasionally and adding more water if needed.

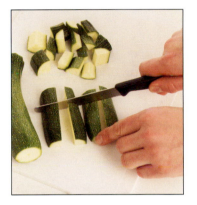

Stir in the tomatoes and season with salt and pepper. Heat until hot and then serve.

Serves 4

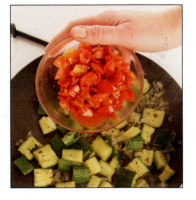

Per serving: 23 Calories, Protein 1 g, Carb 5 g,
Fiber 1 g, Total fat <1 g, Sat fat <1 g, Chol 0 mg,
Sodium 6 mg
Exchanges: 1 Vegetable

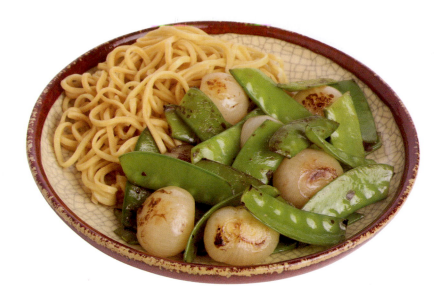

— SNOW PEAS & PEARL ONIONS —

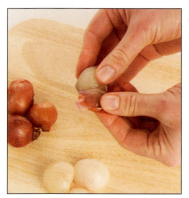

10 oz red or white pearl onions
8 oz snow peas
2 teaspoons canola oil
3 thin slices peeled fresh ginger
salt and freshly ground pepper, to taste

Bring a pot of water to a boil. Add the onions and boil for 4 minutes. Drain and place in cold water until cool and drain again. Cut off stem and root ends and peel off skin.

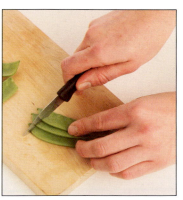

Slice off the pea ends and remove the strings. Heat the oil in a large nonstick skillet or preheated wok over medium heat. Add the ginger and onions and stir-fry for about 3 minutes.

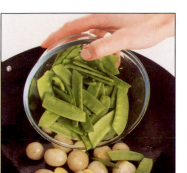

Add the peas and stir-fry for 2 minutes or until the vegetables are crisp-tender. Season with salt and pepper. Remove the ginger slices and serve hot.

Serves 4

Per serving: 77 Calories, Protein 2 g, Carb 12 g, Fiber 2 g, Total fat 5 g, Sat fat <1 g, Chol 0 mg, Sodium 5 mg
Exchanges: 1.5 Vegetable, 0.5 Fat

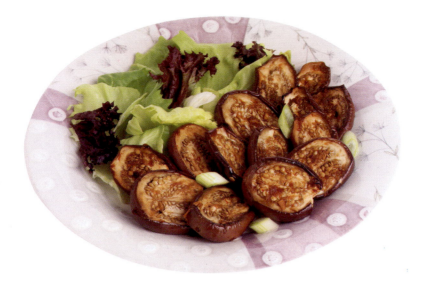

— BAKED ASIAN EGGPLANTS —

about 2 lb Asian-type eggplants (or any long, slender
  eggplant)
1 tablespoon light soy sauce
1 tablespoon sesame oil
1 tablespoon unseasoned rice vinegar
1 teaspoon minced peeled fresh ginger
1 clove garlic, minced
dash of hot pepper sauce or to taste
sliced green onions, for garnish

Preheat oven to 400F (200C). Cut the stem
end off the eggplants. Slice each eggplant
lengthwise into 3 slices.

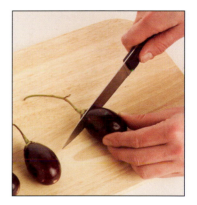

Arrange the slices on a nonstick baking
sheet. Combine the remaining ingredients,
except the onions, in a small bowl and
spoon some over each slice. Bake for 10
minutes.

Turn and spoon the remaining sauce over
the eggplants. Bake for 10 minutes or until
eggplant is tender. Garnish with the onions.
Serve warm or at room temperature.

Serves 4

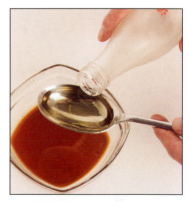

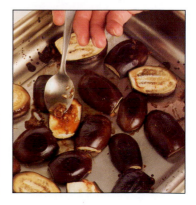

> **Per serving:** 57 Calories, Protein 1 g, Carb 6 g,
> Fiber 2 g, Total fat 4 g, Sat fat <1 g, Chol 0 mg,
> Sodium 228 mg
> **Exchanges:** 1.1 Vegetable, 0.7 Fat

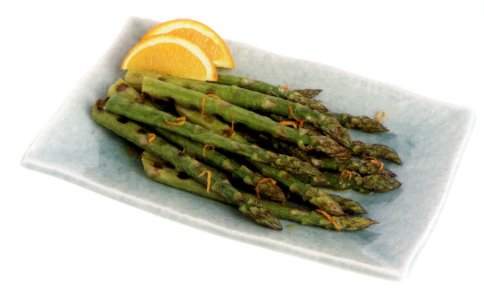

GRILLED ASPARAGUS

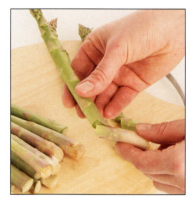

1 lb fresh asparagus
1 tablespoon olive oil
salt and freshly ground pepper, to taste
1 tablespoon orange juice
$^1/_2$ tablespoon balsamic vinegar
1 tablespoon grated orange peel

Preheat a grill or broiler. Snap the tough ends off the asparagus.

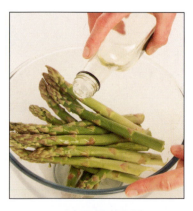

Toss the asparagus with the olive oil. Season with salt and pepper. Arrange the asparagus on the grill rack or broiler pan. Grill until crisp-tender, about 5 minutes, turning once. Toss with the juice, vinegar, and orange peel. Serve hot or at room temperature.

Serves 4

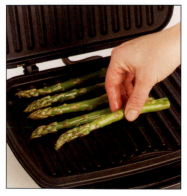

Variation: Grilled Asparagus & Peppers. Substitute 1 yellow, red, or orange bell pepper, cut into thin strips, for half of the asparagus.

Per serving: 65 Calories, Protein 2 g, Carb 6 g, Fiber 3 g, Total fat 3 g, Sat fat <1 g, Chol 0 mg, Sodium 0 mg
Exchanges: 1 Vegetable, 0.7 Fat

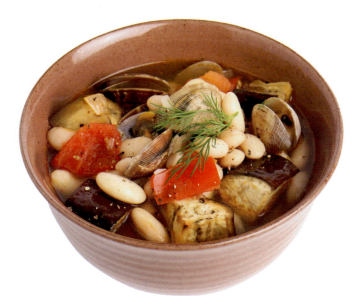

STEAMED CLAMS

1 eggplant, unpeeled, cut into 1-inch pieces
1 tablespoon olive oil
1 shallot, minced
2 cloves garlic, minced
1 cup dry white wine or water
1 (14½-oz) can reduced-fat chicken broth
2 cups chopped Roma tomatoes
1 (15-oz) white beans (navy, Great Northern, or
  cannellini), drained and rinsed
salt, freshly ground black pepper, and hot pepper
  sauce, to taste
48–54 steamer clams, scrubbed
chopped fresh parsley, for garnish

Preheat oven to 425F (220C).

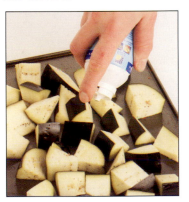

Arrange the eggplant on a large baking sheet. Spray with cooking spray and toss. Bake for 15 minutes, turning once, until almost tender. Heat the oil in a Dutch oven over medium heat. Add the shallot and garlic. Sauté until fragrant. Add the wine and broth and bring to a boil. Stir in the tomatoes, eggplant, and beans. Bring to a boil. Reduce heat and simmer for 5 minutes. Season with salt, pepper, and hot pepper sauce. Increase heat to high and bring back to a boil. Stir in the clams. Cover and cook until the clams open, about 5 minutes.

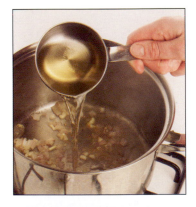

Discard any that remain closed. Divide clams among 6 bowls. Spoon vegetables and broth over clams and sprinkle with parsley.

Serves 6

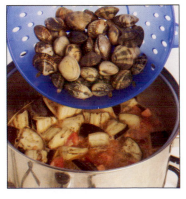

Per serving: 234 Calories, Protein 22 g, Carb 28 g,
Fiber 6 g, Total fat 4 g, Sat fat <1 g, Chol 37 mg,
Sodium 438 mg
Exchanges: 1 Bread/Starch, 2 Lean Meat, 1.5
Vegetable, 1 Fat

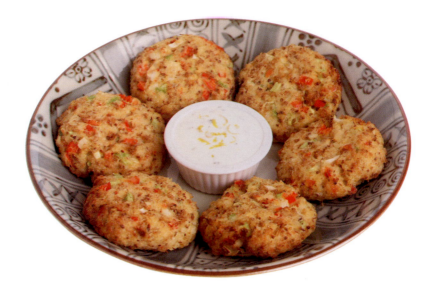

CRAB CAKES

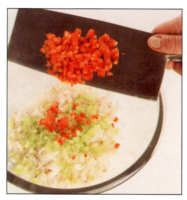

1 lb fresh or frozen thawed crabmeat, picked over to
   remove any shell or cartilage
¹/₄ cup each minced onion and celery
¹/₄ cup minced red bell pepper
1 egg white
¹/₄ cup reduced-fat mayonnaise
1 tablespoon coarse-grain Dijon mustard
1 teaspoon prepared horseradish
¹/₄ cup whole grain cracker crumbs
CHIMICHURRI SAUCE:
¹/₄ cup chopped parsley
2 cloves garlic, minced
1 tablespoon fresh lemon juice
1 teaspoon grated lemon peel
¹/₄ cup reduced-fat mayonnaise
¹/₄ cup plain reduced-fat yogurt

Combine the crabmeat, onion, celery, and
bell pepper in a medium bowl. In another
bowl, lightly beat the egg white. Add the
mayonnaise, mustard, and horseradish. Stir
in the crabmeat mixture and crumbs. Cover
and refrigerate for 30 minutes. To make the
sauce, combine all the ingredients in a small
bowl; set aside. Preheat oven to 425F
(220C). Line a baking sheet with parchment paper. Divide the crabmeat mixture
into 10 equal portions.

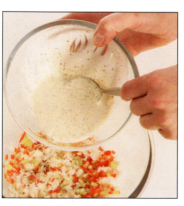

Shape each into a patty and arrange on the
baking sheet. Bake for 15 minutes, until
lightly browned. Serve with the sauce.

Makes 10 crab cakes

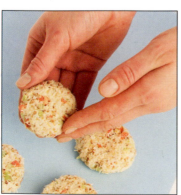

Per crab cake with ¹/₁₀ of sauce: 106 Calories,
Protein 11 g, Carb 4 g, Fiber <1g, Total fat 5 g,
Sat fat 1 g, Chol 36 mg, Sodium 328 mg
Exchanges: 1.3 Very Lean Meat, 1 Fat

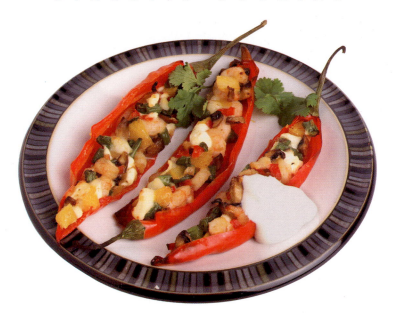

SHRIMP-STUFFED CHILIES

6 large mild fresh chilies such as poblano
3 oz crimini mushrooms, sliced
1/2 red bell pepper, diced
2 cloves garlic, minced
1 cup blanched green beans, chopped into 1/2-inch pieces
8 oz cooked peeled small shrimp
1/2 cup chopped fresh mango
6 oz crumbled soft goat cheese, cut into 4 slices
plain low-fat yogurt, to serve
fresh cilantro leaves, for garnish

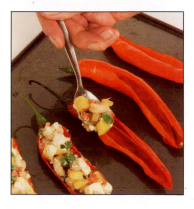

Roast the whole chilies under a preheated broiler or on a grill, until charred on all sides. Place in a self-sealing plastic bag or covered bowl to steam and cool.

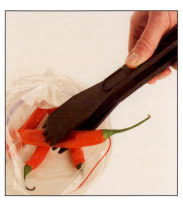

Peel the chilies and cut a slit in the sides to remove the seeds and cores. Preheat oven to 400F (200C). Spray a nonstick baking pan and a nonstick skillet with cooking spray. Add the mushrooms, bell pepper, and garlic to the skillet and cook until softened, stirring occasionally. Stir in the beans, shrimp, mango, and cheese. Place the chilies in the baking pan and spoon in the shrimp mixture. Bake for about 20 minutes or until filling is hot and the cheese softens. Spoon a dollop of yogurt over each chili and garnish with cilantro.

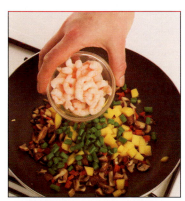

Serves 6

Note: roasted red or green bell peppers can be used instead of poblano chilies.

Per serving: 152 Calories, Protein 14 g, Carb 8 g, Fiber 3 g, Total fat 7 g, Sat fat 4 g, Chol 70 mg, Sodium 396 mg
Exchanges: 1 Very Lean Meat, 1 Lean Meat, 1 Vegetable, 0.8 Fat

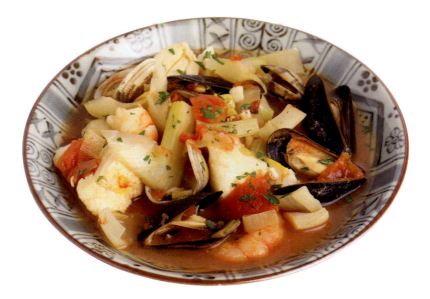

SEAFOOD STEW

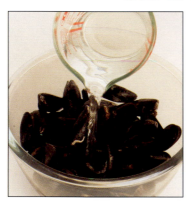

12–16 mussels, scrubbed and beards removed
1 tablespoon olive oil
1 large leek, white part only, finely chopped
1 small white onion, thinly sliced
1 large clove garlic, minced
2 medium fennel bulbs, trimmed and thickly sliced,
   tops chopped and reserved for garnish
1 cup dry white wine or water
1 (14½-oz) can diced tomatoes
3 cups reduced-sodium chicken broth or clam juice
3 cups water
1 (3-inch) strip lemon peel
2 bay leaves and 2 pinches saffron threads
8 oz firm white fish fillets, cut into 1½-inch cubes
12 peeled raw shrimp
12–16 clams, scrubbed
chopped fresh parsley, for garnish
1 cup whole-wheat croutons, to serve

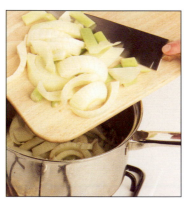

Soak the mussels in cold water for 20 minutes and discard any open shells. Heat the oil in a large saucepan over medium heat. Add the leek, onion, and garlic. Sauté until softened. Stir in the fennel. Add the wine, tomatoes, broth, water, lemon peel, bay leaf, and saffron. Bring to a boil. Reduce heat, cover and simmer for 20 minutes, until vegetables are tender. Bring to a boil. Add the fish and seafood. Cover and boil for 5 minutes, until the clams and mussels open and the fish is cooked through. Discard any shellfish that do not open.

Remove the bay leaves and lemon peel. Divide the stew into bowls. Sprinkle with fennel leaves and parsley. Serve with croutons.

Serves 6

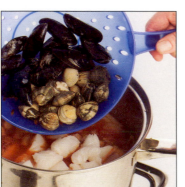

Per serving: 230 Calories, Protein 20 g, Carb 25 g, Fiber 5 g, Total fat 5 g, Sat fat 1 g, Chol 0 mg, Sodium 584 mg
Exchanges: 1.8 Very Lean Meat, 2.4 Vegetable, 1.1 Fat

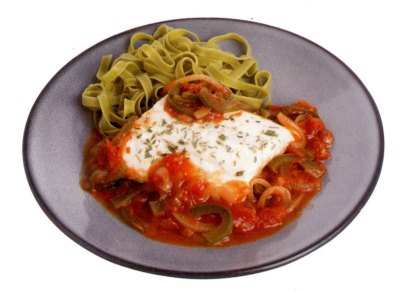

— HALIBUT WITH BELL PEPPERS —

1 tablespoon olive oil
1 small white onion, thinly sliced
1 clove garlic, minced
1 green bell pepper, thinly sliced
1 (14^1/$_2$-oz) can diced tomatoes
4 (6-oz) halibut or cod steaks
1^1/$_2$ teaspoons chopped fresh tarragon or ^{3}/$_4$ teaspoon dried

Heat the oil in a large nonstick skillet over medium heat. Add the onion and garlic and cook until softened, stirring occasionally.

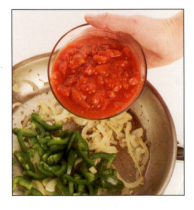

Add the bell pepper, tomatoes with juice, and wine. Bring to a boil. Arrange the halibut over the tomatoes and sprinkle with the tarragon. Reduce heat to low. Cover and simmer until the fish just begins to flake, about 20 minutes, depending on thickness of the fish.

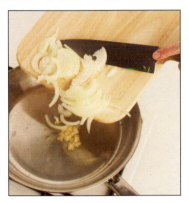

To serve, divide the fish and vegetables among 4 plates.

Serves 4

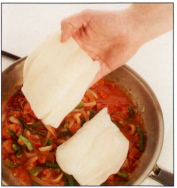

Per serving: 254 Calories, Protein 37 g, Carb 8 g, Fiber 2 g, Total fat 7 g, Sat fat 1 g, Chol 54 mg, Sodium 245mg
Exchanges: 5 Very Lean Meat, 1.6 Vegetable, 0.7 Fat

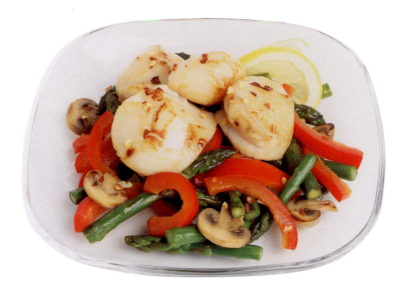

SCALLOP-MUSHROOM STIR-FRY

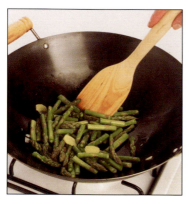

8 oz sea scallops
2 teaspoons canola oil
3 thin slices peeled fresh ginger
1 small clove garlic, minced
8 oz fresh asparagus, cut into 2-inch lengths
1/2 red bell pepper, thinly sliced
3 oz mushrooms, sliced
1 tablespoon fresh lemon juice
hot red pepper flakes, to taste
light soy sauce, to taste
chopped fresh cilantro, for garnish

Cut scallops in half crosswise and slice in half if large; set aside. Heat the oil in a large skillet or wok over high heat.

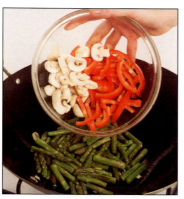

Add the ginger, garlic, and asparagus. Stir-fry for 2–3 minutes. Add the bell pepper and mushrooms. Stir-fry until vegetables are softened, about 2 minutes. Remove vegetables with a slotted spoon. Add the scallops and stir-fry for about 2 minutes or until scallops are opaque. Drizzle lemon juice over the scallops. Return the vegetables to the skillet and season with pepper flakes and soy sauce. Discard the ginger.

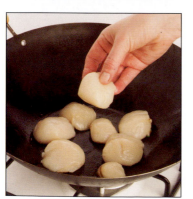

Serve with scallops with the vegetables and garnish with cilantro.

Serves 2

Per serving: 200 Calories, Protein 22 g, Carb 14 g, Fiber 4 g, Total fat 6 g, Sat fat <1 g, Chol 37 mg, Sodium 185 mg
Exchanges: 2.6 Very Lean Meat, 2.1 Vegetable, 0.9 Fat

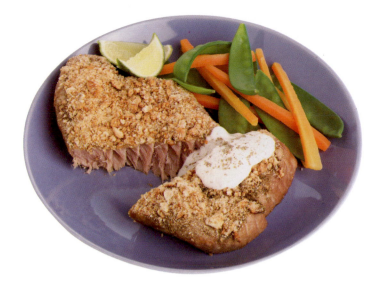

WASABI-GLAZED TUNA STEAKS

4 (about 6-oz) tuna steaks
salt and freshly ground pepper, to taste
¼ cup panko (Japanese bread crumbs)
WASABI SAUCE:
1 tablespoon wasabi powder
1 tablespoon warm water
¼ cup reduced-fat mayonnaise
¼ cup plain, reduced-fat yogurt
2 teaspoons grated peeled fresh ginger
2 teaspoons fresh lemon juice

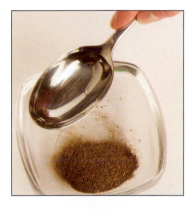

Preheat broiler. To make the wasabi sauce, stir together the wasabi powder and water in a small bowl.

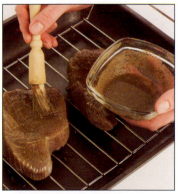

Stir in the mayonnaise, yogurt, ginger, and lemon juice. Remove 2 tablespoons of the mayonnaise sauce and reserve the remaining sauce. Brush half of the wasabi sauce over the tuna. Season the tuna with salt and pepper and place on a rack in a broiler pan. Broil for 10 minutes. Turn and brush the remaining wasabi sauce on the tuna.

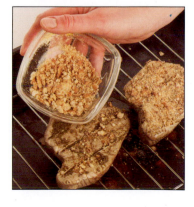

Sprinkle with the panko, pressing it in lightly. Broil for 5 minutes, until only a thin line in the center of the tuna is still pink. Serve with the remaining wasabi sauce.

Serves 4

Per serving: 292 Calories, Protein 43 g, Carb 6 g, Fiber <1 g, Total fat 9 g, Sat fat 1 g, Chol 6 mg, Sodium 137 mg
Exchanges: 3.9 Lean Meat, 1 Fat

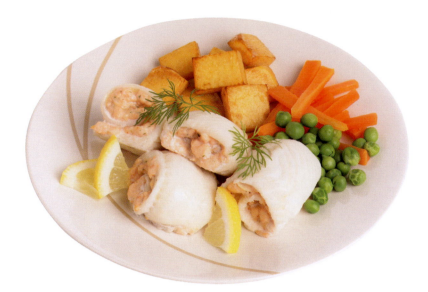

FLOUNDER & SALMON MOUSSE

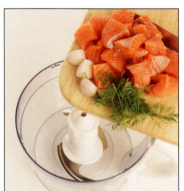

8 oz salmon fillets, any bones removed, cut into
  chunks
1 shallot, minced
2 teaspoons fresh dill or 1 teaspoon dried
2 egg whites
1/4 teaspoon salt
freshly ground pepper, to taste
dash of hot pepper sauce
4 flounder, sole, or trout fillets
fresh dill sprigs, for garnish
lemon wedges, to serve

In a food processor, combine the salmon,
shallot, and dill. Pulse until mixture is
pureed.

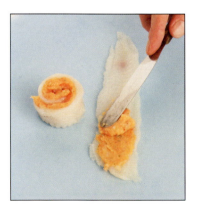

Add the egg whites and season with salt,
pepper, and hot pepper sauce. Pulse until
combined. Divide the salmon mixture into
4 equal portions. Lay the flounder out on a
work surface. Spread each flounder with
salmon mixture and roll up jelly-roll
fashion. Place a steamer basket over boiling
water. Arrange flounder rolls in steamer
basket; season with salt and pepper.

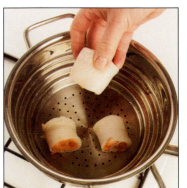

Steam until fish is firm to the touch and
cooked through, about 15 minutes. Transfer
the rolls to serving plates. Garnish with dill
sprigs and serve with lemon wedges.

Serves 4

Per serving: 238 Calories, Protein 43 g, Carb <1 g,
Fiber <1 g, Total fat 5 g, Sat fat 1 g, Chol 0 mg,
Sodium 584 mg
Exchanges: 4.6 Very Lean Meat, 1.5 Lean Meat

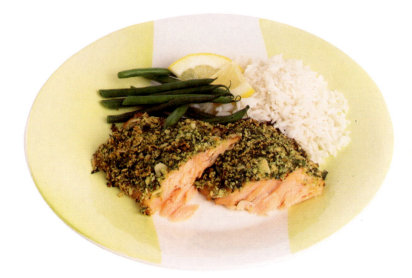

NUT-CRUSTED SALMON

¹/₂ cup sliced almonds
2 tablespoons chopped fresh parsley
1 teaspoon grated lemon peel
1 tablespoon reduced-fat mayonnaise
1 tablespoon coarse-grain mustard
1 tablespoon dry white wine
4 (6-oz) salmon fillets
lemon wedges, to serve

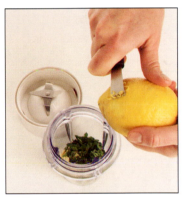

Preheat oven to 425F (220C). Spray a non-stick baking sheet with cooking spray. Combine the almonds, parsley, and lemon peel in a mini food processor or blender. Process until almonds are finely chopped.

Combine the mayonnaise, mustard, and wine in a small bowl. Brush over the top of the salmon. Using your fingers, press the almond mixture over the salmon. Arrange the salmon on the prepared baking sheet.

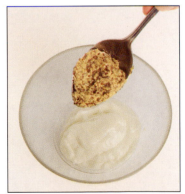

Bake for 20 minutes or until the salmon just begins to flake. Serve with lemon wedges.

Serves 4

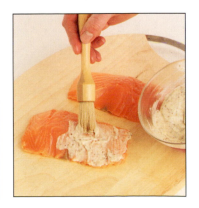

Per serving: 379 Calories, Protein 38 g, Carb 4 g, Fiber 2 g, Total fat 22 g, Sat fat 2 g, Chol 96 mg, Sodium 158 mg
Exchanges: 0.5 Very Lean Meat, 5 Lean Meat, 2.3 Fat

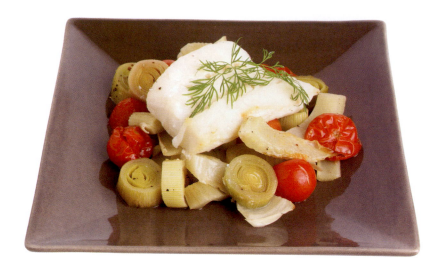

BAKED FISH WITH FENNEL

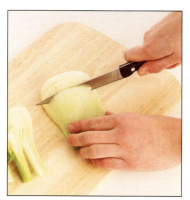

1 fennel bulb
1 cup sliced leeks (white and pale green parts)
2 cups cherry or grape tomatoes, halved if large
1 clove garlic, minced
2 teaspoons olive oil
salt and freshly ground pepper, to taste
4 (4–6-oz) fish fillets, such as halibut, cod, or
  haddock
4 teaspoons fresh lemon juice

Preheat oven to 425F (220C). Cut the stalks from the fennel bulb. Cut the bulb in half, remove the hard core, and slice cross-wise into $1/4$-inch thick slices.

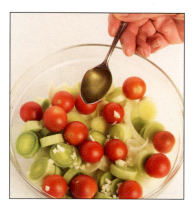

Coarsely chop the fennel leaves. Combine the leeks, sliced fennel, tomatoes, garlic and oil in a bowl. Season with salt and pepper. Arrange in a baking dish large enough to hold the fish in one layer. Arrange the fillets over the vegetable mixture in a single layer. Drizzle the lemon juice over the fish and sprinkle with the fennel leaves.

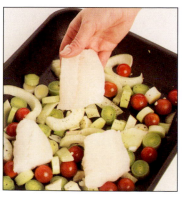

Bake for 20 minutes or until the fish just begins to flake when tested with a fork and the vegetables are softened.

Serves 4

Per serving: 210 Calories, Protein 26 g, Carb 15 g, Fiber 4 g, Total fat 6 g, Sat fat 1 g, Chol 36 mg, Sodium 109 mg
Exchanges: 3.4 Very Lean Meat, 2.6 Vegetables

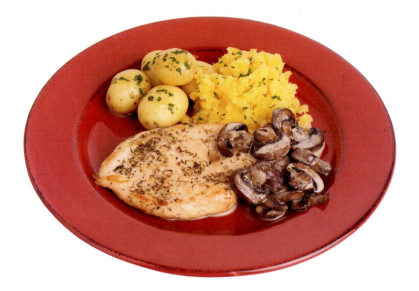

— CHICKEN WITH MARSALA —

4 (4–6-oz) boneless, skinless chicken breast halves
1 tablespoon olive oil
1 shallot, minced
4 oz fresh mushrooms, sliced
1 teaspoon dried thyme
salt and freshly ground pepper, to taste
1/2 cup Marsala wine
3 tablespoons fat-free half-and-half

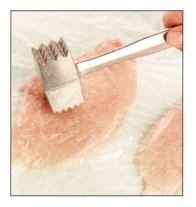

Rinse the chicken; pat dry with paper towels. Place between 2 pieces of plastic wrap. Pound lightly with a meat mallet to flatten to about 1/2 inch thick; set aside. Heat the oil in a large skillet over medium heat. Add the shallot. Cook for 1 minute.

Add the mushrooms and cook until the mushrooms are softened and begin to brown, about 5 minutes. Transfer the mixture to a bowl and set aside. Add the chicken to the skillet, in batches, and increase heat to medium-high. Cook until browned. Sprinkle the chicken with the thyme and season with salt and pepper. Add the Marsala and reduce heat to medium-low. Cover and cook for 10 minutes, until the chicken is cooked through and juices run clear. Transfer to a serving platter and keep warm.

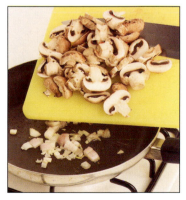

Add the mushroom mixture back to the skillet. Add the half-and-half, stir to combine, and heat until hot; do not boil. Spoon over chicken breasts and serve.

Serves 4

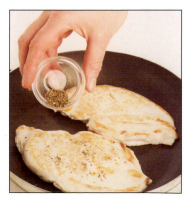

Per serving: 211 Calories, Protein 27 g, Carb 5 g, Fiber <1g, Total fat 5 g, Sat fat 1 g, Chol 66 mg, Sodium 78 mg
Exchanges: 4 Very Lean Meat/Protein, 2 Fat

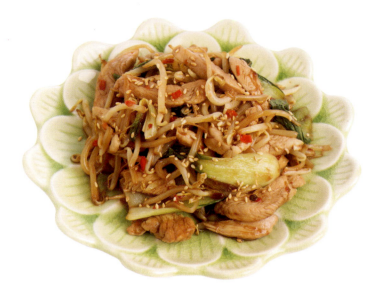

CHICKEN STIR-FRY

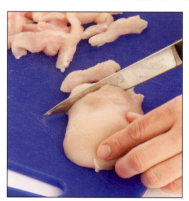

2 (4-oz) boneless, skinless, chicken breast halves
2 teaspoons grated peeled fresh ginger
1 clove garlic, minced
2 tablespoons ponzu sauce
1 tablespoon sesame oil
6 green onions (green and white parts), cut into
    1-inch pieces
1 medium jalapeño chili, seeded, minced
4 baby bok choy, chopped into 1–2-inch pieces
1 lb bean sprouts
1 tablespoon sesame seeds, toasted

Rinse the chicken; pat dry with paper towels. Cut the chicken into thin strips.

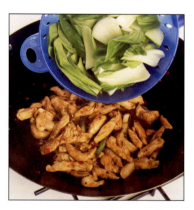

Transfer to a bowl. Stir in the ginger, garlic, and sauce; let stand at room temperature for 20 minutes, stirring occasionally. Heat the sesame oil in a preheated wok or large skillet over high heat. Add the green onions and stir-fry until softened. Add the chicken and stir-fry until no longer pink in the centers. Add the chili and bok choy; stir until softened, about 2 minutes. Add the bean sprouts and stir-fry until bean sprouts are hot. Sprinkle with sesame seeds and serve.

Serves 2–3

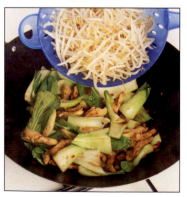

Note: ponzu sauce is soy sauce seasoned with citrus. Use 1 tablespoon light soy sauce and 1 tablespoon lemon juice as an alternative.

Per serving: 296 Calories, Protein 41 g, Carb 28 g, Fiber 12 g, Total fat 5 g, Sat fat 1 g, Chol 66 mg, Sodium 584 mg
Exchanges: 4 Very Lean Meat/Protein, 5 Vegetable, 0.5 Fat

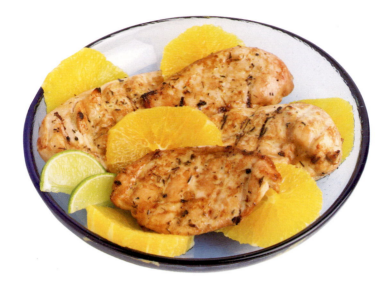

CHICKEN IN CITRUS MARINADE

1–2 oranges
4 (4–6-oz) boneless, skinless chicken breast halves
1/4 cup orange juice
1 tablespoon soy sauce
2 tablespoons olive oil
1 clove garlic, crushed
1/2 teaspoon dried thyme
salt and freshly ground pepper, to taste

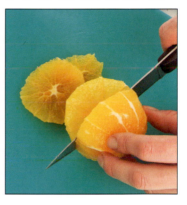

Peel the oranges, remove the white pith, and cut crosswise into slices. Set aside. Rinse the chicken; pat dry with paper towels. Arrange in a glass dish or place in a self-sealing plastic bag.

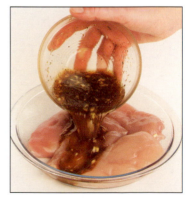

Combine the remaining ingredients in a small bowl, except oranges. Pour over the chicken and turn to coat. Let marinate for 30 minutes at room temperature or 1 hour in the refrigerator. Preheat grill or broiler. Remove the chicken from marinade, discarding the marinade.

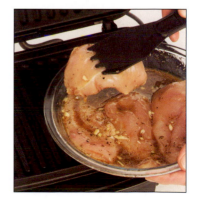

Place the chicken on the grill rack. Grill for 15 minutes, until chicken is cooked through, turning once. Serve with the oranges.

Serves 4

Per serving: 209 Calories, Protein 27 g, Carb 5 g, Fiber <1 g, Total fat 8 g, Sat fat 1 g, Chol 66 mg, Sodium 303 mg
Exchanges: 4 Very Lean Meat/Protein, 1 Fat

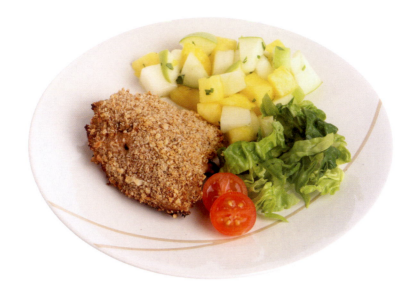

NUT-CRUSTED CHICKEN

4 (about 4-oz) boneless, skinless chicken thighs
1 cup buttermilk
¹/4 cup coarsely ground almonds
2 tablespoons dried bread crumbs
4 teaspoons five-spice powder
salt and freshly ground pepper, to taste
fruit salsa, to serve (optional)

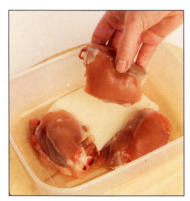

Rinse the chicken; pat dry with paper towels. Place the buttermilk in a shallow dish. Add the chicken, turning to coat. Let marinate for 30 minutes at room temperature or 1 hour in the refrigerator.

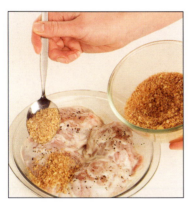

Preheat oven to 400F (200C). Combine the almonds, bread crumbs, and five-spice powder. Drain the chicken and season with salt and pepper. Coat with the almond mixture. Place the chicken on a nonstick baking sheet. Bake until the crust is browned and the chicken is cooked through, about 20 minutes.

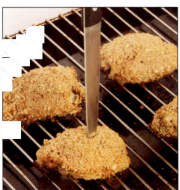

If the chicken is not browned, broil for a few minutes, watching carefully to avoid burning the coating. Serve with fruit salsa (if liked).

Serves 4

Per serving: 316 Calories, Protein 23 g, Carb 7 g, Fiber <1 g, Total fat 21 g, Sat fat 5 g, Chol 98 mg, Sodium 180 mg
Exchanges: 3 Lean Meat/Protein, 2.5 Fat

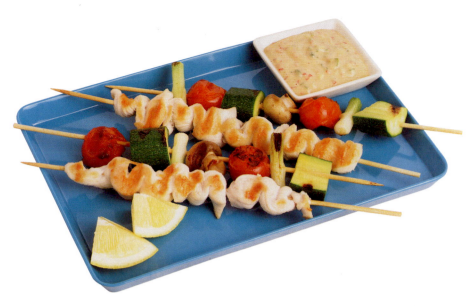

CHICKEN-VEGETABLE KEBOBS

4 (4–6-oz) boneless, skinless chicken breasts, cut
  into thin strips
2 zucchini, cut into 2-inch pieces
6 green onions, white part only, cut into 1-inch
  pieces
6 cherry tomatoes
12 button mushrooms
salt and freshly ground pepper, to taste
PEANUT SAUCE:
1/4 cup creamy peanut butter
about 1/4 cup reduced-sodium chicken broth
2 tablespoons unseasoned rice vinegar
1 tablespoon soy sauce
1 small red hot chili, seeded and minced, or to taste
1 tablespoon minced green onion tops
1 tablespoon grated peeled fresh ginger

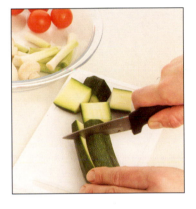

Soak 8–10 bamboo skewers, depending on
length, in water for 30 minutes. Preheat a
grill or broiler. To make the sauce, stir
together the peanut butter and broth until
smooth. Stir in remaining ingredients.
Arrange the chicken strips on skewers, using
about 3 strips per skewer. Alternate vegetables on remaining skewers. Season the
kebobs with salt and pepper and place the
on the grill rack. Grill for 20 minutes,
turning as needed, until chicken is browned
and cooked through and vegetables are
crisp-tender.

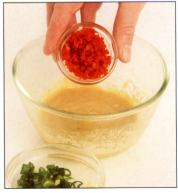

Transfer the kebobs to a serving platter.
Drizzle with the peanut sauce or serve on
the side.

Serves 4

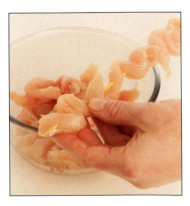

Per serving: 215 Calories, Protein 31 g, Carb 7 g,
Fiber 2 g, Total fat 7 g, Sat fat 1 g, Chol 66 mg,
Sodium 293 mg
Exchanges: 4 Very Lean Meat/Protein,
1 Vegetable, 1 Fat

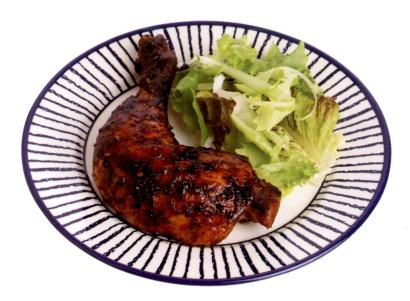

CHERRY-CHIPOTLE CHICKEN

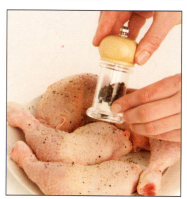

4 chicken legs
salt and freshly ground pepper, to taste
CHERRY-CHIPOTLE SAUCE:
$1/2$ canned chipotle chili in adobo sauce, or to taste
$1/3$ cup morello cherry fruit spread
about $1/4$ cup reduced-sodium chicken broth
2 tablespoons unseasoned rice vinegar
$1/2$ teaspoon dried oregano

Rinse the chicken; pat dry with paper towels. Season with salt and pepper and set aside. Remove the stem and seeds from the chili.

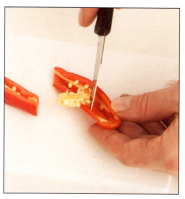

Transfer the chili, fruit spread, and broth to a blender. Blend until pureed. Add the vinegar and oregano. Preheat a grill or broiler. Place the chicken on the grill rack. Grill for 10 minutes; turn and brush with sauce. Grill for 5 minutes; turn and brush other side with sauce. Grill until chicken is cooked through, the juice runs clear when a skewer is inserted into the thickest part of the meat, and the internal temperature reaches 170F (75C).

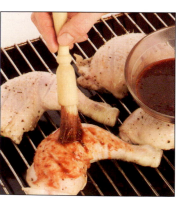

Serves 4

Note: remove skin before cooking—otherwise sauce is lost.

> **Per serving:** 392 Calories, Protein 31 g, Carb 18 g, Fiber <1 g, Total fat 20 g, Sat fat 6 g, Chol 139 mg, Sodium 160 mg
> **Exchanges:** 1 Other Carbs/Sugar, 4.5 Lean Meat/Protein, 2 Fat

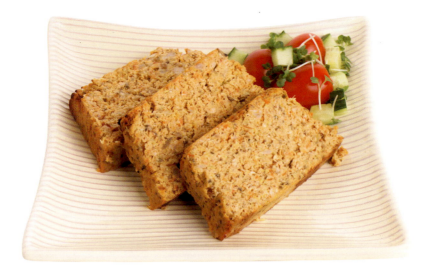

TURKEY-ARTICHOKE LOAF

1 tablespoon olive oil
4 oz fresh mushrooms, chopped
1/2 cup shredded carrot
1 medium white onion, chopped
1 clove garlic, minced
1 (14-oz) can artichoke hearts, drained
1 lb extra-lean ground turkey
1/2 pound Italian turkey sausage, casing removed
1/2 cup tomato sauce
salt and freshly ground pepper, to taste

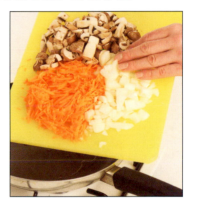

Preheat the oven to 350F (180C). Grease a 9 x 5-inch loaf pan. Heat the oil in a large skillet over medium heat. Add the mushrooms, carrots, onion, and garlic.

Cook until softened, remove from skillet, and cool. Transfer the mushroom mixture to a food processor. Add the artichoke hearts and pulse until finely chopped. Add the turkey, turkey sausage, and tomato sauce to the food processor and pulse until combined. Transfer the mixture to the prepared pan and smooth the top. Bake for 1 hour or until the top is browned and an instant-read thermometer inserted in the center registers 170F (75C).

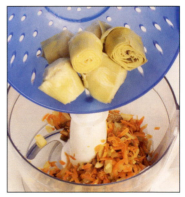

Let cool in the pan for 10 minutes before slicing. Serve warm or cold.

Serves 6

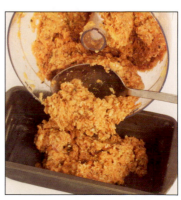

Per serving: 264 Calories, Protein 23 g, Carb 14 g, Fiber 4 g, Total fat 13 g, Sat fat 4 g, Chol 89 mg, Sodium 852 mg
Exchanges: 3 Lean Meat/Protein, 2 Vegetable, 1 Fat

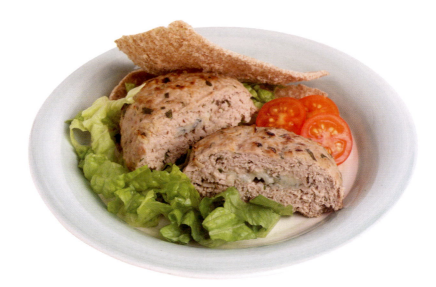

— TURKEY CHEESE BURGERS —

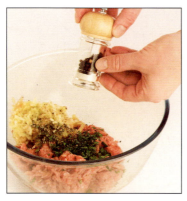

1 lb very lean ground turkey
1 cup shredded apple
1 teaspoon chopped fresh sage or 1/2 teaspoon dry
1 tablespoon chopped fresh parsley
dash of freshly ground nutmeg
1/2 teaspoon salt or to taste
freshly ground pepper, to taste
2–4 oz creamy blue cheese
4 whole-wheat pita bread halves, lettuce, and
    tomatoes slices to serve

Add the turkey, apple, sage, parsley, nutmeg, salt, and pepper in a bowl and mix until combined.

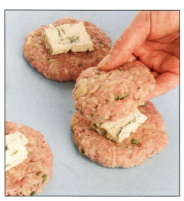

Shape the turkey mixture into 8 thin patties. Place one-fourth of the cheese in the center of 4 patties. Top with remaining patties, sealing the edges. Preheat a grill or broiler. Grill for 10 minutes, or until the turkey is cooked through and a thermometer inserted sideways into the burgers registers 165F (75C).

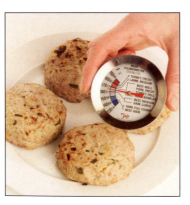

Insert into pita halves with lettuce and tomatoes (if using).

Serves 4

Per serving: 364 Calories, Protein 37 g, Carb 39 g, Fiber 6 g, Total fat 7 g, Sat fat 3 g, Chol 81 mg, Sodium 882 mg
Exchanges: 2 Bread/Starch, 3.6 Very Lean Meat/Protein, 0.6 Fat

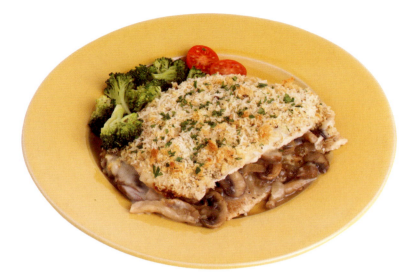

TURKEY MUSHROOM BAKE

6 (3–4-oz) turkey cutlets
salt and freshly ground pepper, to taste
1 tablespoon olive oil
10 oz fresh mixed mushrooms, sliced
$^1/_2$ cup chopped onion
1 clove garlic, minced
2 teaspoons fresh thyme or $^1/_2$ teaspoon dried
1 teaspoon fresh chopped oregano or $^1/_2$ teaspoon dried
1$^1/_2$ cups skim milk or fat-free half-and-half
1$^1/_2$ tablespoons cornstarch
$^1/_2$ cup dry white wine
$^1/_8$ teaspoon freshly grated nutmeg
1 tablespoon low-sodium bread crumbs mixed with 1
   tablespoon freshly grated Parmesan cheese
2 tablespoons chopped fresh parsley, for garnish

Preheat oven to 350F (180C).

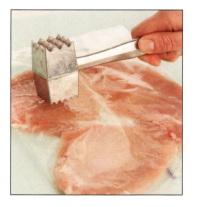

Place the turkey between 2 sheets of plastic wrap. Pound with a meat mallet until $^1/_4$ inch thick. Season with salt and pepper. Heat the oil in a nonstick skillet over medium heat. Cook the turkey until no longer pink. Set aside. Add the mushrooms, onion, and garlic to the skillet. Cook until softened. Layer the turkey and mushroom mixture in a medium oval baking dish, sprinkling the turkey with the herbs. Whisk a little of the milk with the cornstarch in a saucepan. Whisk in the remaining milk, wine, and nutmeg. Cook over medium heat, stirring, until thickened.

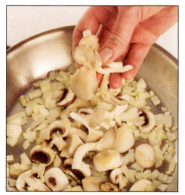

Pour over the turkey and mushrooms. Sprinkle with the crumb mixture. Bake for 30 minutes, until hot and bubbly. Garnish with the parsley.

Serves 6

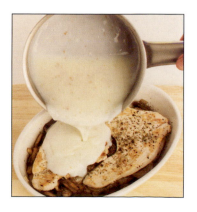

Per serving: 220 Calories, Protein 23 g, Carb 11 g,
Fiber 1 g, Total fat 9 g, Sat fat 2 g, Chol 57 mg,
Sodium 219 mg
Exchanges: 2.6 Very Lean Meat, 0.6 Vegetable,
1.6 Fat

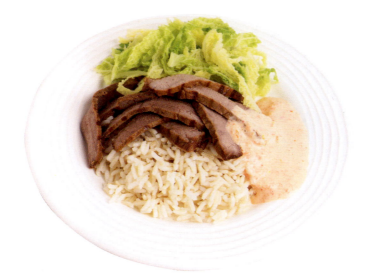

— FLANK STEAK & RED PEPPER —

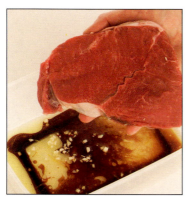

2 tablespoons olive oil
2 tablespoons lemon juice
grated peel of ¹/₂ lemon
1 tablespoon soy sauce
1 teaspoon sugar or 1 (¹/₄-teaspoon) packet Splenda®
  no calorie sweetener
1 clove garlic, minced
1 (about 1¹/₂-lb) beef flank or round steak, trimmed
RED PEPPER SAUCE:
1 red bell pepper
¹/₄ cup reduced-fat mayonnaise
¹/₄ cup plain nonfat yogurt
1 clove garlic, minced
grated peel of ¹/₂ lemon
dash of hot pepper sauce
salt and freshly ground pepper, to taste

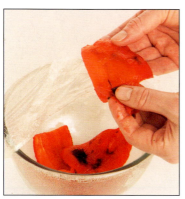

Combine the oil, lemon juice, peel, soy sauce, sugar, and garlic in a plastic lidded container. Add the steak and turn to coat. Seal and refrigerate for at least 2 hours. Preheat a grill or broiler. To make the sauce, grill the bell pepper on all sides until charred. Place in a covered bowl for 10 minutes to cool. Peel and cut into strips. Add the bell pepper, mayonnaise, yogurt, garlic, and lemon peel to a food processor and pulse until combined. Season with hot pepper sauce, salt, and pepper. Remove the steak from the marinade and pat dry.

Grill, turning as needed, for 20 minutes, or until medium-rare to medium. Cut into thin slices. Serve with the sauce.

Serves 6

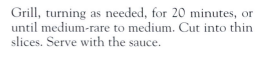

Per serving: 350 Calories, Protein 32 g, Carb 7 g,
Fiber 1 g, Total fat 20 g, Sat fat 7 g, Chol 5 mg,
Sodium 32 mg
Exchanges: 4.5 Very Lean Meat/Protein, 0.3
Vegetable, 3.6 Fat

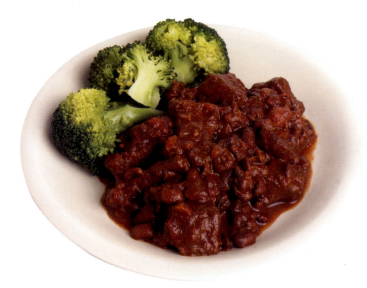

CHILI WITH BLACK BEANS

1 tablespoon olive oil
1 lb beef round or chuck steak, cut into 1-inch cubes
1 medium onion, chopped
1 clove garlic, minced
1 oz bittersweet chocolate, finely chopped
1 tablespoon mild or medium chili powder
1 teaspoon ground cumin
1/4 teaspoon ground cinnamon
dash of ground cloves
1 bay leaf
1/2 teaspoon dried oregano
2 cups reduced-sodium beef broth
2 cups water
1 (14 1/2-oz) can diced tomatoes
2 (15-oz) cans black beans, drained
salt and freshly ground pepper, to taste

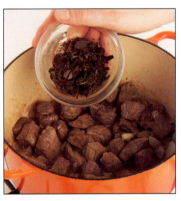

Heat the oil in a large pot over medium heat. Add the beef, in batches, and cook until browned. Stir in the onion and garlic. Add the chocolate, spices, herbs, broth, and water. Cover and simmer until beef is very tender, stirring occasionally, about 1 hour. Stir in the tomatoes and beans.

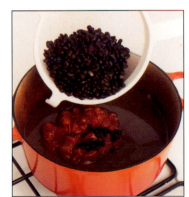

Bring to a boil, reduce heat, and simmer for about 10 minutes to allow the flavors to blend. Season with salt and pepper.

Makes 8 (1-cup) servings

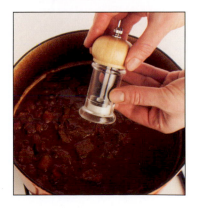

Per cup: 229 Calories, Protein 19 g, Carb 22 g, Fiber 7 g, Total fat 9 g, Sat fat 3 g, Chol 34 mg, Sodium 560 mg
Exchanges: 1 Bread/Starch, 2 Lean Meat/Protein, 1 Vegetable, 1 Fat

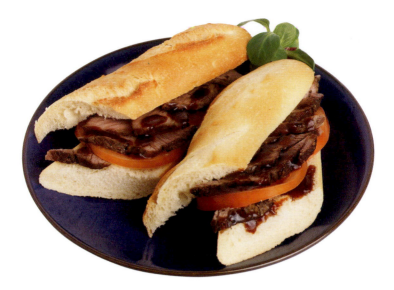

SLOW-ROASTED BEEF

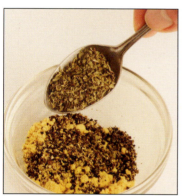

1^1/$_2$ tablespoons coarsely ground or cracked black
   pepper
1 tablespoon dry mustard
1 teaspoon dried thyme
salt, to taste
1 (about 3-lb) rolled beef roast
barbecue sauce (optional)

Preheat the oven to 325F (165C). In a small
bowl, combine the pepper, mustard, thyme,
and salt.

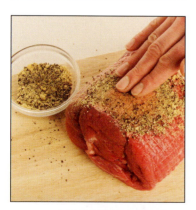

Rub the spice mixture over the beef. Add 2
cups of water to a roasting pan, place the
beef on a rack in the pan, and cover. Roast
for 3^1/$_2$ hours or until very tender (the
center of the beef should register 325F
(160C) on an instant-read thermometer).
Slice the roast on the diagonal or shred for
sandwiches and serve with barbecue sauce,
if desired.

Serves 12

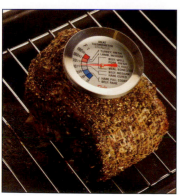

Note: leftovers can be frozen in serving-size
portions for up to 1 month.

Per serving without sauce: 357 Calories, Protein
24 g, Carb <1 g, Fiber <1 g, Total fat 24 g, Sat fat
9 g, Chol 108 mg, Sodium 67 mg
Exchanges: 4 Lean Meat/Protein, 2 Fat

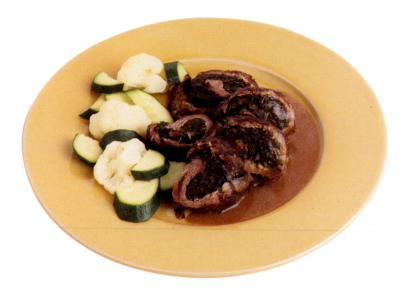

STEAK WITH SPINACH & CHEESE

1 (about 2-lb) boneless beef round steak, trimmed
²/₃ cup red wine
²/₃ cup water
1 teaspoon cornstarch mixed with 2 tablespoons water
STUFFING:
2 (9-oz) packages fresh spinach
freshly ground nutmeg, to taste
salt and freshly ground pepper, to taste
¹/₄–¹/₂ cup crumbled blue cheese

Preheat oven to 350F (180C). Place the steak between 2 sheets of plastic wrap. Pound with a meat mallet to ¹/₄-inch thickness, being careful not to tear the meat.

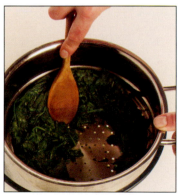

Cook the spinach in a small amount of boiling water in a large pot over medium-high heat until just wilted. Drain, cool, and squeeze out any moisture. Combine the spinach, nutmeg, salt, and pepper in a medium bowl. Spread the spinach over the beef, leaving about 2 inches uncovered at one end. Sprinkle the cheese over the spinach. Roll up, jelly-roll style, and tie with kitchen twine. Place on a rack in a roasting pan. Add the wine and water to the pan. Cover and roast for 2 hours, until the steak is very tender. Remove the steak to a plate.

Place the pan over medium heat and stir the cornstarch mixture into the pan juices. Cook, stirring, until slightly thickened. Cut the steak into crosswise slices and serve with the sauce.

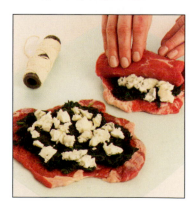

Serves 8

Per serving: 254 Calories (1061 kilojoules),
Protein 27 g, Carb 2 g, Fiber 1 g, Total fat 13 g,
Sat fat 6 g, Chol 48 mg, Sodium 258 mg
Exchanges: 3.7 Lean Meat/Protein, 1 Fat

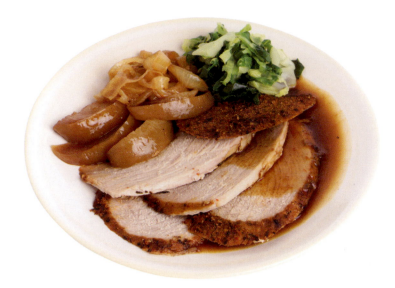

JERK PORK ROAST

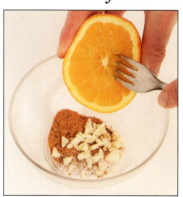

1 tablespoon salt-free jerk seasoning
2 cloves garlic, minced
1/4 cup fresh orange juice
1/4 cup fresh lemon juice
1/2 teaspoon salt
freshly ground pepper, to taste
1 (2-lb) pork roast
3 medium apples
1 large white onion, sliced
1/2 cup white wine

Combine the jerk seasoning, garlic, juices, salt, and pepper in a small bowl.

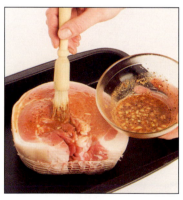

Preheat oven to 350F (180C). Rub the jerk mixture over the pork and let stand for 20 minutes. Cut the apples into quarters, core, and slice. Arrange the apples and onion in the bottom of a Dutch oven. Add the wine and place the pork in the pan. Cover and roast for 2 hours or until the pork is very tender. Transfer the pork to a cutting board and keep warm.

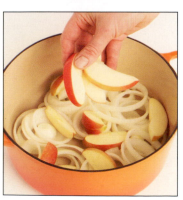

Place the pan over medium-high heat and boil to reduce cooking juices to a sauce. Slice the pork and serve with the apples, onion, and sauce.

Serves 8

> **Per serving:** 349 Calories, Protein 31 g, Carb 15 g, Fiber 3 g, Total fat 16 g, Sat fat 6 g, Chol 92 mg, Sodium 408 mg
> **Exchanges:** 4 Lean Meat/Protein, 1 Fruit, 1 Fat

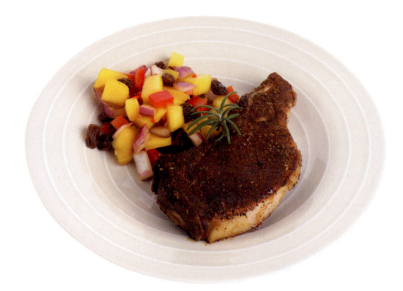

PORK WITH MANGO CHUTNEY

1 tablespoon mild chili powder
1 teaspoon ground cumin
$^1/_2$ teaspoon ground thyme
$^1/_2$ teaspoon salt, or to taste
freshly ground pepper, to taste
4 (1-inch-thick) pork chops, trimmed of extra fat
MANGO CHUTNEY:
1 mango, cubed
2 tablespoons zante currants
2 tablespoons diced red bell pepper
1 tablespoon minced jalapeño chili, or to taste
2 tablespoons minced red onion
1 tablespoon unseasoned rice vinegar
2 teaspoons grated peeled fresh ginger
2 teaspoons brown sugar
$^1/_4$ teaspoon salt, or to taste

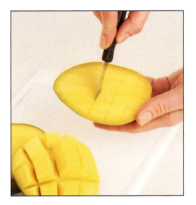

To make the chutney, combine the mango with the currants, bell pepper, chili, onion, vinegar, ginger, sugar, and salt in a medium bowl. Cover and let stand at room temperature for flavors to blend. Transfer to a saucepan and heat just until hot. Remove from heat and keep warm. Preheat a grill or broiler. Combine the chili powder, cumin, thyme, salt, and pepper in a small bowl. Rub on all sides of the pork. Let stand at room temperature for 20 minutes.

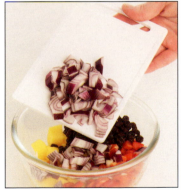

Grill for 15 minutes, until the centers are just barely pink and interior temperature is at least 150F (65C). Serve with the chutney.

Serves 4

Per serving: 210 Calories, Protein 20 g, Carb 16 g, Fiber 2 g, Total fat 7 g, Sat fat 2 g, Chol 57 mg, Sodium 511 mg
Exchanges: 2.5 Lean Meat/Protein, 0.5 Fruit, 0.5 Vegetable

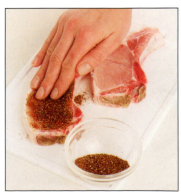

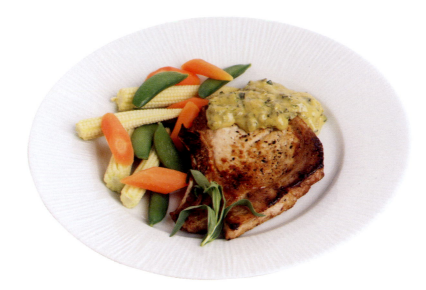

— CUTLETS WITH HERB SAUCE —

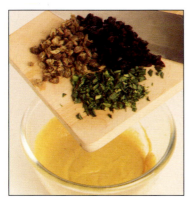

4 (4–6-oz) pork cutlets
salt and freshly ground black pepper, to taste
1 tablespoon olive oil
HERB SAUCE:
1½ tablespoons Dijon mustard
1 tablespoon unseasoned rice vinegar
½ teaspoon sugar
2 tablespoons olive oil
1 tablespoon minced Kalamata olives
1 teaspoon capers, drained and minced
1 tablespoon fresh minced tarragon or
    1½ teaspoons dried

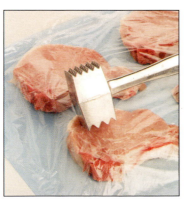

To make the sauce, combine the mustard, vinegar, and sugar in a bowl. Gradually whisk in the oil. Add the olives, capers, and tarragon. Set aside. Place the pork between 2 sheets of plastic wrap. Pound with a meat mallet until about ¼-inch thick. Season the pork with salt and pepper. Heat the oil in a large skillet over medium heat. Add the pork and sauté until browned and cooked through, turning as needed.

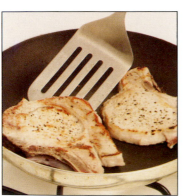

Transfer the cutlets to serving plates and accompany with the sauce.

Serves 4

Per serving: 251 Calories, Protein 22 g, Carb 2 g, Fiber <1 g, Total fat 17 g, Sat fat 4 g, Chol 58 mg, Sodium 224 mg
Exchanges: 3 Very Lean Meat/Protein, 3 Fat

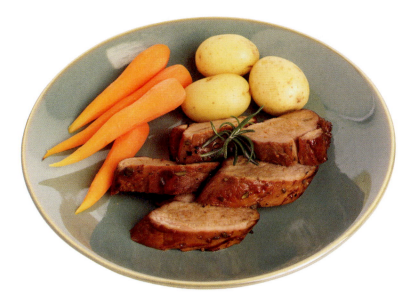

— TENDERLOIN & TANGERINE —

1 (about 1-lb) pork tenderloin
salt and freshly ground pepper, to taste
rosemary sprig, for garnish (optional)
TANGERINE GLAZE:
1/2 cup tangerine juice
2 tablespoons balsamic vinegar
1 teaspoon chopped fresh rosemary, plus extra for
  garnish (optional)

To make the glaze, simmer the tangerine
juice, vinegar, and rosemary until reduced
by half.

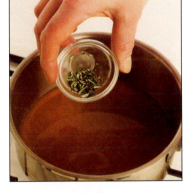

Preheat a grill or boiler. Remove the silver-
skin from the pork with a sharp, thin knife.
Season with salt and pepper. Grill the pork
until browned on underside, about 10
minutes. Turn and brush with glaze. Grill
for about 10 minutes, turn, and brush
with the glaze. Continue grilling until
cooked through and the center of the pork
registers 160F (70C) on an instant-read
thermometer.

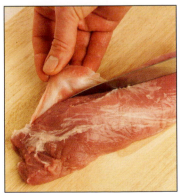

Transfer to a cutting board and cut into thin
slices. To serve, garnish with rosemary
(if using).

Serves 4

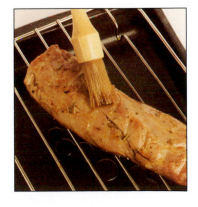

> **Per serving:** 154 Calories, Protein 24 g, Carb 4 g,
> Fiber <1 g, Total fat 4 g, Sat fat 1 g, Chol 74 mg,
> Sodium 59 mg
> **Exchanges:** 3 Very Lean Meat/Protein, 1 Fat

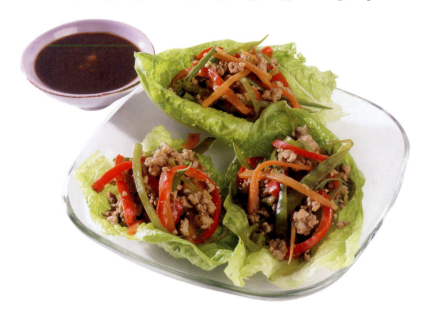

SOUTHEAST ASIAN PORK CUPS

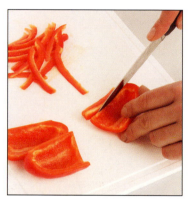

1 tablespoon canola oil
1 lb lean ground pork
6 green onions, white and green parts, minced
1 clove garlic, minced
1 cup shredded carrot
1 red bell pepper, julienned
1 cup julienned snow peas (about 20 peas)
2 teaspoons soy sauce, or to taste
cupped lettuce leaves, to serve
fresh cilantro leaves, to serve
DIPPING SAUCE:
2 tablespoons hoisin sauce
1 tablespoon unseasoned rice vinegar
1 tablespoon sesame oil
1 teaspoon minced peeled fresh ginger

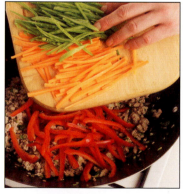

1 clove garlic, minced
chili sauce, such as sriracha, to taste

Heat the oil in a large skillet or wok over medium heat. Add the pork, onions, and garlic and cook, stirring to break up meat, until the pork is no longer pink. Add the carrot, bell pepper, and snow peas. Stir-fry for 1 minute. Stir in the soy sauce. Spoon pork mixture into lettuce leaves. Top with cilantro leaves.

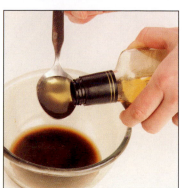

Combine the ingredients for the dipping sauce in a small serving dish and serve with the stir-fry.

Serves 4

Per serving: 266 Calories, Protein 26 g, Carb 13 g, Fiber 3 g, Total fat 12 g, Sat fat 2 g, Chol 71 mg, Sodium 353 mg
Exchanges: 0.5 Bread/Starch, 4.5 Very Lean Meat/Protein, 1 Vegetable, 1 Fat

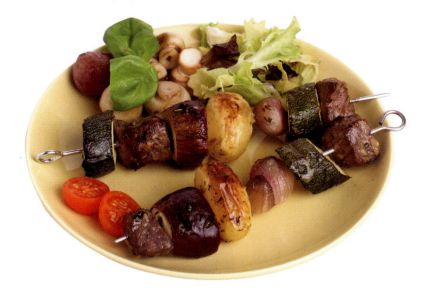

LAMB KEBOBS

1 lb lean leg of lamb, cut into 2-inch pieces
8 fingerling or baby potatoes
8 zucchini, cut into 2-inch pieces
8 small cipolline or other small onions, peeled
8 button mushrooms
2 Japanese eggplants, cut into 2-inch pieces
basil leaves, for garnish
MARINADE:
2 tablespoons each lemon juice and olive oil
1 tablespoon grated lemon peel
1 clove garlic, minced
1 teaspoon each dried mint and dried rosemary

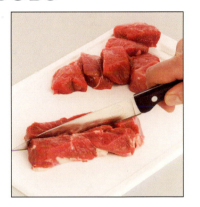

Combine the marinade ingredients in a large plastic self-sealing bag. Add the lamb, turn to coat, and refrigerate for 2–8 hours.

Steam the potatoes and zucchini for 10 minutes, until just tender. Set aside. (If using baby potatoes bigger than the lamb pieces halve after precooking.) Bring a pan of water to a boil, add the onions, and boil for 5 minutes, until just tender. Remove with a slotted spoon. Preheat a grill or broiler. Remove the lamb from the marinade, reserving the marinade, and pat dry with paper towels. Thread onto skewers with the vegetables. Brush with reserved marinade.

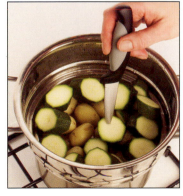

Grill until the lamb is cooked as desired, about 15 minutes for medium, and the vegetables are tender. Garnish with mint.

Serves 4

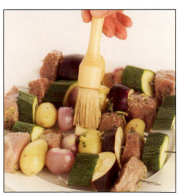

Per serving: 348 Calories, Protein 30 g, Carb 31 g, Fiber 11 g, Total fat 12 g, Sat fat 3 g, Chol 72 mg, Sodium 196 mg
Exchanges: 0.5 Bread/Starch, 3 Very Lean Meat/Protein, 4 Vegetable, 2 Fat

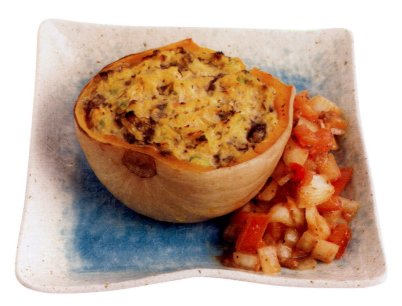

STUFFED SQUASH

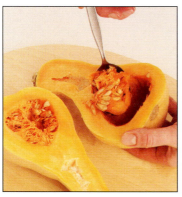

1 (about 12–16-oz) butternut or acorn squash
6 oz fresh button mushrooms, chopped
1/2 cup (4 oz) mashed silken tofu or ricotta cheese
1/2 cup grated reduced-fat soy or regular cheddar cheese
1 tablespoon minced fresh basil or 1 teaspoon dried
1 tablespoon finely chopped chives or spring onion tops
dash of hot pepper sauce
salt and freshly ground black pepper, to taste
FRESH TOMATO SAUCE:
2 Italian plum tomatoes, diced
1 tablespoon diced onion
1 tablespoon sun-dried or regular tomato puree
1/2 teaspoon white wine vinegar
1 teaspoon chopped fresh oregano or 1/2 teaspoon dried
salt and freshly ground black pepper, to taste

Preheat the oven to 400F (200C).

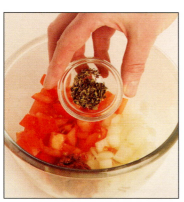

Cut the squash in half and remove the seeds. Steam over boiling water for 15 minutes, until tender. Let cool. Remove the flesh with a spoon, leaving a 1/2-inch shell. Mash the squash and set aside. To make the sauce, combine all the ingredients in a small bowl; reserve. Heat a skillet over medium heat. Spray with cooking spray and add the mushrooms; cook until softened. Combine the tofu, squash, mushrooms, cheese, basil, chives, pepper sauce and black pepper in a bowl. Spoon the cheese mixture into the squash halves and place in a baking dish.

Bake for 20 minutes, until filling is set and tops are browned. Spoon the sauce onto plates and top with the squash.

Serves 2

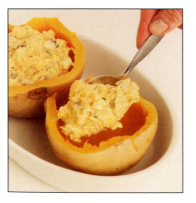

Per serving: 211 Calories, Protein 19 g, Carb 13 g, Fiber 3 g, Total fat 11 g, Sat fat 5 g, Chol 123 mg, Sodium 333 mg
Exchanges: 1.3 Very Lean Meat/Protein, 1.7 Lean Meat, 1 Vegetable, 1.2 Fat

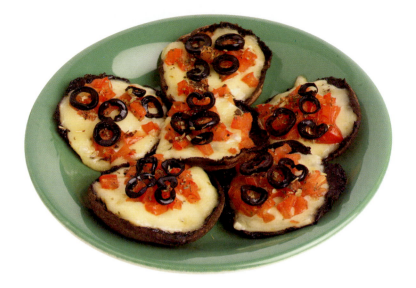

PORTOBELLO PIZZAS

8 portobello mushrooms
4 slices reduced-sodium, part-skim mozzarella cheese
4 Roma tomatoes, chopped
1 tablespoon dried basil
1 teaspoon dried oregano
freshly ground black pepper, to taste
2 tablespoons sliced pitted kalamata olives

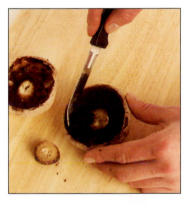

Preheat oven to 425F (220C). Wipe mushrooms with a damp paper towel. Remove gills with a grapefruit spoon or small knife. Cut off the stems flush with the caps. Place the mushrooms, gill sides down on a rack, on a baking sheet.

Spray tops with cooking spray. Roast for 10 minutes. Turn mushrooms gill sides up. Place a slice of cheese on each mushroom. Top with the tomatoes.

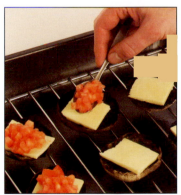

Sprinkle with the herbs and pepper. Divide the olives among the pizzas. Bake for 5–8 minutes or until the cheese is melted.

Makes 8 mini pizzas

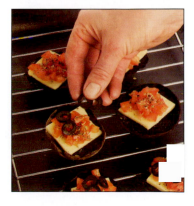

Per 2 pizzas: 133 Calories, Protein 11 g, Carb 9 g, Fiber 2 g, Total fat 6 g, Sat fat 3 g, Chol 15 mg, Sodium 77 mg
Exchanges: 1.1 Lean Meat, 1.5 Vegetable, 0.6 Fat

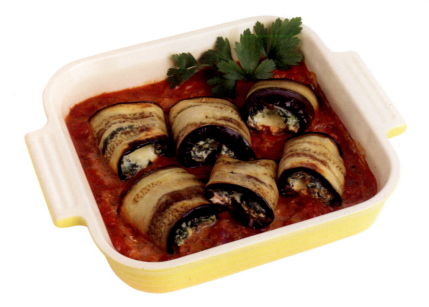

EGGPLANT ROLL-UPS

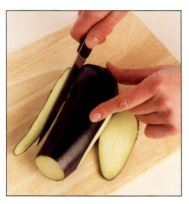

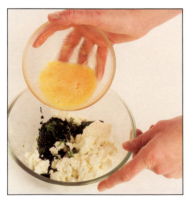

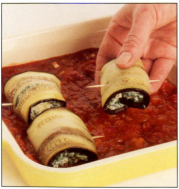

1 large or 2 medium eggplant, stem and tip removed
1 (10-oz) package frozen chopped spinach
1 lb reduced-fat ricotta cheese
1 egg, beaten
2 teaspoons chopped fresh basil or 1 teaspoon dried
1 teaspoon chopped fresh oregano or ¹/₂ teaspoon dried
freshly ground black pepper, to taste
1 cup shredded reduced-fat mozzarella cheese
EASY TOMATO SAUCE:
1 (14¹/₂-oz) can diced tomatoes
1 (8-oz) can Italian-seasoned tomato sauce
1 small white onion, minced
1 clove garlic, minced
2 teaspoons chopped fresh basil or 1 teaspoon dried
freshly ground black pepper, to taste

Preheat the oven to 350F (180C).

Spray a nonstick baking sheet with cooking spray. Remove the peel from two sides of the eggplant. Slice lengthwise into 8 slices. Arrange in a single layer on the baking sheet. Bake for 10 minutes, until tender. Cook the spinach according to package directions. Cool and drain. With your hands, squeeze the moisture from the spinach. Combine with the ricotta cheese, egg, herbs, and pepper in a bowl. Divide the cheese mixture among the slices and sprinkle with mozzarella. Roll up, jelly-roll style. Secure with wooden picks.

Mix the sauce ingredients and pour into a baking dish. Place the rolls on top. Bake until bubbly and filling begins to brown. Remove wooden picks and serve.

Serves 4, 2 rolls each

Per serving: 330 Calories, Protein 26 g, Carb 24 g, Fiber 7 g, Total fat 15 g, Sat fat 9 g, Chol 105 mg, Sodium 580 mg
Exchanges: 3 Lean Meat, 3.5 Vegetable, 1.7 Fat

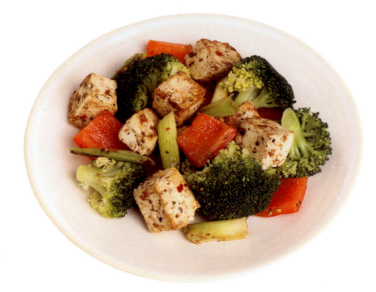

BROCCOLI-TOFU STIR-FRY

8 oz firm tofu
8 oz broccoli florets
1 teaspoon Thai seasoning
2 teaspoons toasted sesame oil
1/2 red bell pepper, cut into 1-inch squares
4 green onions, white and green parts, cut into
   1-inch lengths
1 tablespoon tamari sauce or to taste

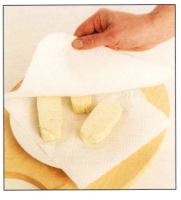

Cut the tofu into 3 slices. Place between paper towels and place a flat pan with a weight on it to press out the excess water. Let stand for about 10 minutes.

Meanwhile, steam the broccoli over boiling water until crisp-tender. Cut the tofu into cubes. Sprinkle with the Thai seasoning and toss to coat. Heat the oil in a large nonstick skillet over medium heat. Add the bell pepper and onions; stir-fry for 2 minutes.

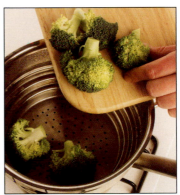

Add the tofu, tamari sauce, and broccoli and stir-fry for another 2 minutes. Serve immediately.

Serves 2

Per serving: 190 Calories, Protein 13 g, Carb 16 g,
Fiber 6 g, Total fat 10 g, Sat fat 1 g, Chol 0 mg,
Sodium 496 mg
Exchanges: 2.4 Very Lean Meat, 2.6 Vegetable,
2.1 Fat

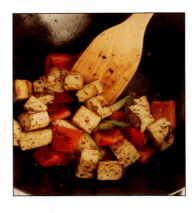

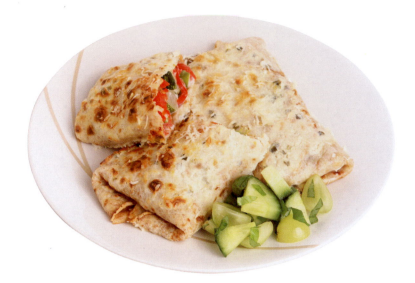

— VEGETABLE STUFFED CREPES —

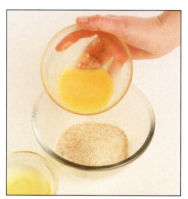

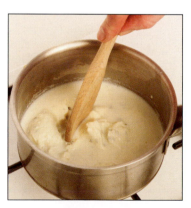

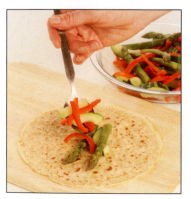

¹/₂ cup each all-purpose flour and whole-wheat flour
pinch of salt
1 egg, plus 2 egg whites
1¹/₂ cups water or skim milk
FILLING:
1 cup light cream cheese with garlic and onion (if
   herbed cheese not available, stir in 1 teaspoon
   minced garlic and 1 tablespoon minced green onion)
about ¹/₂ cup skim milk
12 asparagus spears, steamed until crisp-tender
¹/₂ red bell pepper, cut into thin strips and steamed
   until crisp-tender
1 small yellow summer squash, cut into thin strips
   and steamed until crisp-tender
2 tablespoons freshly grated Parmesan cheese

Preheat oven to 400F (200C).

Whisk the crepe ingredients together until smooth. Chill for 30 minutes. Heat a 7–8-inch nonstick pan over medium-high heat. Spray with cooking spray. Add 3 tablespoons batter. Swirl to coat pan. Cook until slightly browned on bottom, turn and cook for 30 seconds. Repeat with remaining batter. Spray a baking dish with cooking spray. Heat the cheese and milk in a saucepan over low heat, stirring. Add more milk if needed to make a thin sauce. Divide the vegetables among the crepes. Spoon half the sauce over the vegetables. Fold into parcels and place seam side down in the

baking dish. Spoon over the remaining sauce and sprinkle with Parmesan. Bake for 15 minutes, until cheese melts and filling is hot.

Serves 6

Per serving: 206 Calories, Protein 11 g, Carb 21 g, Fiber 3 g, Total fat 8 g, Sat fat 5 g, Chol 57 mg, Sodium 307 mg
Exchanges: 0.9 Bread/Starch, 0.7 Very Lean Meat/Protein, 0.7 Vegetables, 1.5 Fat

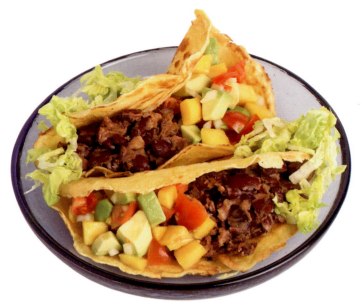

VEGETARIAN TACOS

1 small avocado, diced
1 medium tomato, diced
$^1/_2$ cup diced mango
2 tablespoons minced onion
1 tablespoon fresh lime juice
2 cups cooked or canned pinto, kidney, or black
  beans with some liquid
$^1/_2$ teaspoon mild ground chile
$^1/_4$ teaspoon ground cumin
$^1/_4$ teaspoon ground coriander
4 corn tortillas
shredded lettuce, to serve

Combine the avocado, tomato, mango, onion, and lime juice in a small bowl.

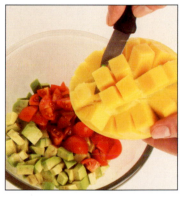

Spray a nonstick skillet with cooking spray. Add the beans with about 2 tablespoons cooking liquid or water. Heat until hot, mashing some of the beans and stirring in the liquid. Stir in the spices.

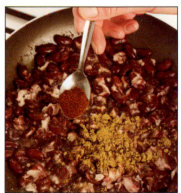

Heat the tortillas in a dry skillet until warmed. Fill the tortillas with the beans and avocado mixture. Top with the lettuce.

Serves 4

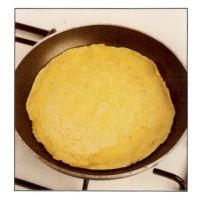

Per serving: 265 Calories, Protein 9 g, Carb 41 g,
Fiber 12 g, Total fat 9 g, Sat fat 1 g, Chol 0 mg,
Sodium 473 mg
Exchanges: 2 Bread/Starch, 0.5 Fruit,
0.4 Vegetable, 1.5 Fat

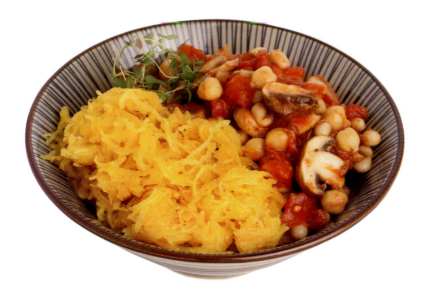

TWO-BEAN SPAGHETTI SQUASH

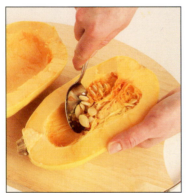

1 (about 3-lb) spaghetti squash, cut in half
TWO-BEAN SAUCE:
1 tablespoon olive oil
1 cup chopped onion
2 cloves garlic, minced
4 oz fresh mushrooms, sliced
1 (14$^1/_2$-oz) can diced tomatoes
1 (8-oz) can no-salt added tomato sauce
1$^3/_4$ cups cooked or canned without salt garbanzo
  beans, drained and rinsed
1$^3/_4$ cups cooked or canned without salt cannelini,
  pinto, or black beans, drained and rinsed
1 teaspoon dried basil
$^1/_2$ teaspoon dried oregano
hot pepper sauce, to taste
salt and freshly ground pepper, to taste

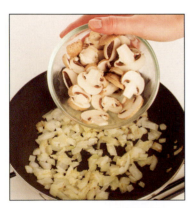

Remove the seeds from the spaghetti squash, cook, and separate into strands (page 45). Heat the oil in a large saucepan over medium heat. Add the onion and garlic and cook until softened, stirring occasionally. Add the mushrooms and cook until softened, stirring occasionally. Add the tomatoes and tomato sauce. Cover and simmer for 10 minutes, until the onion is almost tender. Stir in the beans and herbs. Simmer, covered, for 20 minutes to combine the flavors, adding a little water if the sauce becomes too thick.

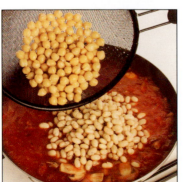

Season with hot pepper sauce, salt, and pepper. Spoon the spaghetti squash into 8 pasta bowls. Top with the sauce and serve.

Serves 8

Per serving: 145 Calories, Protein 8 g, Carb 20 g, Fiber 6 g, Total fat 3 g, Sat fat <1 g, Chol 0 mg, Sodium 78 mg
Exchanges: 0.8 Bread/Starch, 0.7 Very Lean Meat/Protein, 1.5 Vegetable, 0.4 Fat

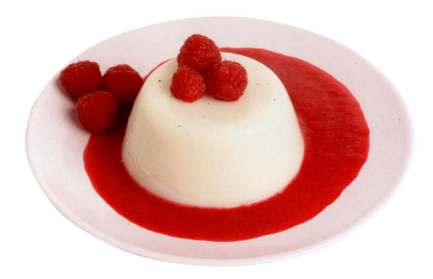

CAFFE LATTÉ PANNA COTTA

$1/2$ cup medium-roast coffee beans
2 cups 2% milk
1 ($1/4$-oz) envelope plain gelatin powder
2 tablespoons cold water
$1/4$ cup sugar
1 teaspoon vanilla extract
2 cups fresh raspberries

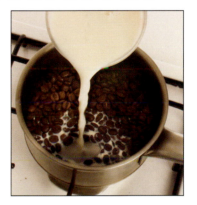

Add the coffee beans to a heavy saucepan over medium-low heat. Heat for about 5 minutes, stirring occasionally, until slightly oily. Add the milk and heat, stirring, until hot. Turn off heat and let stand for 30 minutes.

Sprinkle the gelatin over the water and let stand for 10 minutes to soften. Either remove the coffee beans with a slotted spoon or pour through a strainer. Add the gelatin to the milk in the saucepan and stir until dissolved. Stir in the sugar and vanilla. Pour into 4 (about $1/2$-cup) molds. Refrigerate until firm. Add 1 cup of the raspberries to a blender or food processor. Process until pureed. Unmold the panna cotta by loosening the edges with a knife and dipping the mold into hot water for a few seconds.

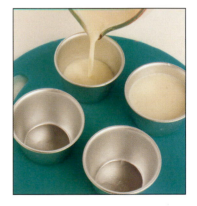

Turn out on dessert plates. Spoon the sauce around the panna cotta and top with the remaining raspberries.

Serves 4

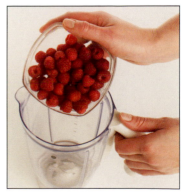

Per serving: 149 Calories, Protein 6 g, Carb 26 g, Fiber 4 g, Total fat 3 g, Sat fat 1 g, Chol 10 mg, Sodium 65 mg
Exchanges: 0.7 Other Carbs/Sugar, 0.5 Fruit, 0.5 Milk, 0.5 Fat

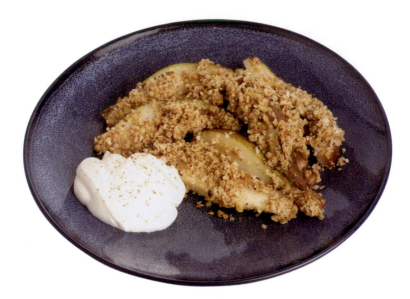

FRESH PEAR CRISP

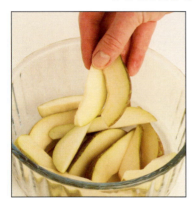

4 cups sliced pears
1 tablespoon lemon juice
2 tablespoons granulated sugar
1/2 cup rolled oats
2 tablespoons chopped hazelnuts
1 tablespoon whole-wheat flour
1/2 teaspoon ground cinnamon
1/4 cup packed light brown sugar
3 tablespoons cold no-trans fat margarine or butter,
   cut into pieces
plain Greek yogurt, to serve (optional)

Preheat oven to 350F (180C). Toss the
pears with the lemon juice and sugar.
Arrange in an 8-inch baking dish.

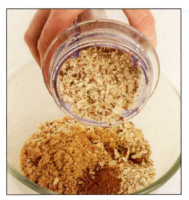

Combine the oats, hazelnuts, flour, cinnamon, and sugar in a medium bowl. Using a
pastry blender or 2 knives, cut the margarine into the oat mixture until crumbly.

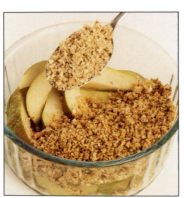

Cover the pears with the oat mixture and
press down. Bake for 30 minutes, until bubbly
and fruit is tender. Serve with yogurt, if liked.

Serves 8

Per serving: 185 Calories, Protein 2 g, Carb 33 g,
Fiber 4 g, Total fat 6 g, Sat fat <1 g, Chol 0 mg,
Sodium 39 mg
Exchanges: 0.3 Bread/Starch, 0.5 Other
Carbs/Sugar, 1.3 Fruit, 1 Fat

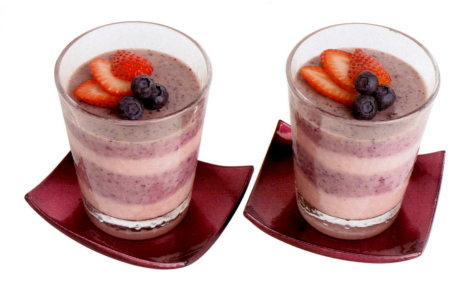

BERRY BAVARIAN

1¹/₂ cups sliced strawberries, pureed
2 tablespoons Splenda® Granular no-calorie sweetener
1 tablespoon sugar
2 tablespoons fresh lemon juice
2 tablespoons grated lemon peel
1¹/₂ cups blueberries, pureed
2 (¹/₄-oz) envelopes plain gelatin powder softened in
    ¹/₄ cup water
1 cup 2% milk
1 cup plain low-fat yogurt
4 strawberry fans and a few blueberries, for garnish

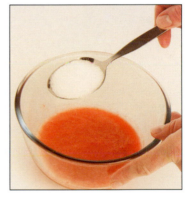

Combine the strawberries, 1 tablespoon Splenda®, ¹/₂ tablespoon sugar, 1 tablespoon lemon juice, and 1 tablespoon lemon peel.

In another bowl, mix the blueberries with the remaining Splenda®, sugar, lemon juice and peel. Heat the milk and gelatin over low heat, stirring, until dissolved. Whisk in the yogurt. Stir half of the yogurt mixture (about 1 cup plus 2 tablespoons) into the strawberry mixture and the other half into the blueberry mixture. Refrigerate for 30 minutes, until beginning to set.

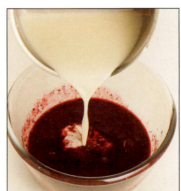

Spoon alternate layers of the semi-set berry mixtures into 4 glasses. Arrange a strawberry fan and a few blueberries on the top. Refrigerate for 1 hour, until completely set.

Serves 4

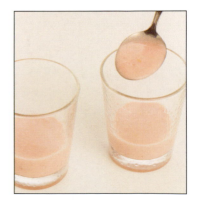

Per serving: 156 Calories, Protein 9 g, Carb 26 g, Fiber 4 g, Total fat 2 g, Sat fat 1 g, Chol 8 mg, Sodium 84 mg
Exchanges: 1 Fruit, Milk, Skim 0.6

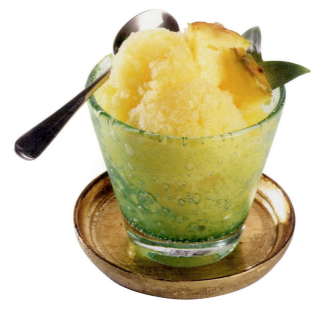

PINEAPPLE-TANGERINE SORBET

1 small to medium pineapple
2 tablespoons sugar
1 cup fresh tangerine juice
1 tablespoon mandarin liqueur or orange liqueur
  (optional)

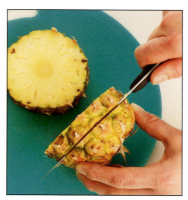

Cut the green top and base off of the pineapple. Cut into slices crosswise, remove the skin and any eyes.

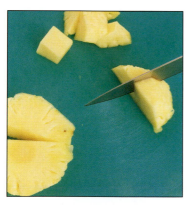

Core and then cut into chunks. Process in a food processor or blender until pureed. Measure 1½ cups. Stir the sugar into the juice until dissolved. Stir in the pineapple and liqueur (if using). Cover and refrigerate until chilled.

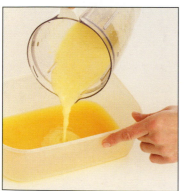

Pour into an ice cream maker. Freeze according to manufacturer's directions.

Makes 6 (¹/2-cup) servings

Per serving: 62 Calories, Protein <1 g, Carb 14 g, Fiber <1 g, Total fat <1 g, Sat fat 0 g, Chol 0 mg, Sodium 1 mg
Exchanges: 0.6 Fruit

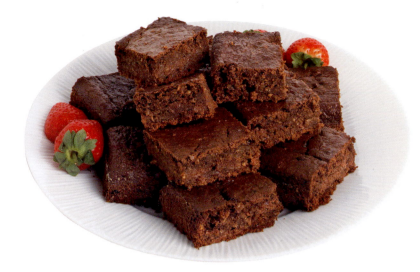

— CHOCOLATE-CHERRY BARS —

1 1/2 cups skim milk
2/3 cup rolled oats
1/3 cup high fiber cereal
1 cup whole-wheat flour
2 teaspoons baking powder
1/8 teaspoon salt
1/2 cup chopped dried cherries
6 oz semisweet chocolate chips, melted
1/4 cup no-trans fat margarine or butter, melted
2/3 cup packed light brown sugar
1 egg
1 ripe banana, mashed
2 teaspoons vanilla extract

Preheat oven to 350F (180C).

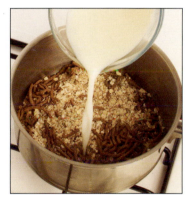

Spray a nonstick 12 x 9-inch baking pan with cooking spray. Combine the milk, oats, and cereal in a saucepan over medium-low heat. Heat, stirring, until hot. Remove from the heat and stand until warm. Mix together the flour, baking powder, and salt in a bowl. Add the cherries and stir to coat. In another bowl, beat together the chocolate, margarine, sugar, egg, banana, and vanilla. Add the cereal mixture to the chocolate mixture and beat until combined. Stir in the dry ingredients. Pour into the prepared pan.

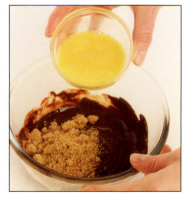

Bake for 25 minutes, until the center is still slightly soft but the edges spring back when pressed. Cool completely and cut into squares.

Makes 16 squares

Per square: 180 Calories, Protein 3 g, Carb 30 g, Fiber 3 g, Total fat 6 g, Sat fat 2 g, Chol 0 mg, Sodium 110 mg
Exchanges: 0.5 Bread/Starch, 0.9 Other Carbs/Sugar, 1 Fat

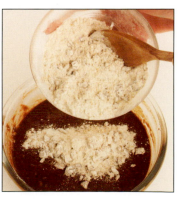

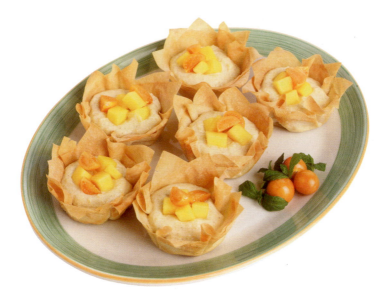

MANGO MOUSSE CUPS

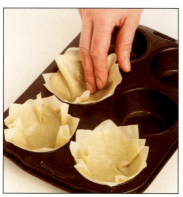

6 sheets phyllo pastry dough, thawed if frozen
3 tablespoons no-trans fat margarine or butter, melted
1/2 cup ricotta cheese
1 tablespoon honey
1 mango, peeled, seeded, and chopped
1/2 teaspoon ground allspice

Preheat oven to 400F (200C). Spray 6 muffin cups with cooking spray. Lightly brush one sheet of phyllo with margarine (keep remaining sheets covered).

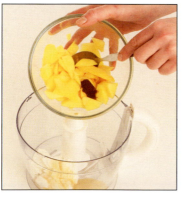

Top with another phyllo sheet and brush with margarine. Cut into 6 (4-inch) squares. Repeat with remaining phyllo and margarine. Stack 3 squares together, rotating corners so they do not overlap. Press each stack into a prepared muffin cup. Bake for 10 minutes or until golden and crispy. Cool on a wire rack. Add the ricotta and honey to a food processor or blender; pulse until combined. Add the mango (reserving a little for garnish) and allspice and pulse until pureed. Refrigerate until chilled.

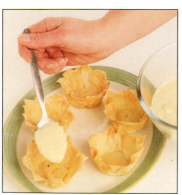

Carefully transfer the phyllo cups to dessert plates. Divide the mango mixture among the cups. Garnish with the reserved mango and serve immediately.

Serves 6

Per serving: 158 Calories, Protein 4 g, Carb 18 g, Fiber 1 g, Total fat 8 g, Sat fat 2 g, Chol 6 mg, Sodium 74 mg
Exchanges: 1.3 Fat

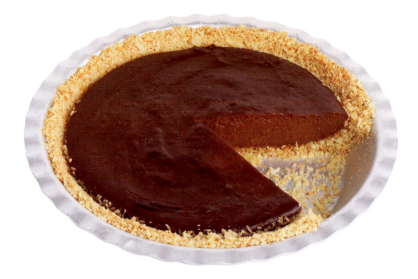

— NUT-CRUST CHOCOLATE PIE —

NUT CRUST:
$1/4$ cup ($1^{1}/_{2}$ oz) slivered almonds
$3/4$ cup all-purpose flour
1 tablespoon powdered sugar
3 tablespoons olive oil
FILLING:
2 tablespoons cornstarch
$1/4$ cup Splenda® Granular no calorie sweetener
2 cups 2% milk
3 oz semisweet chocolate, chopped
2 teaspoons vanilla extract
whipping cream, whipped to serve (optional)

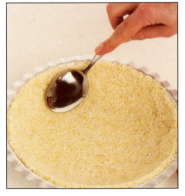

Preheat oven to 400F (200C). Spray a 9-inch pie pan with cooking spray.

Pulse the almonds in a food processor or blender until finely chopped. Combine the almonds, flour, sugar, oil and about 2 tablespoons water in a medium bowl. Press into the bottom and sides of the pie pan. Bake for 10–12 minutes, until lightly browned. Cool on a wire rack. Combine the cornstarch, Splenda®, and $1/4$ cup of the milk to make a paste in a medium saucepan. Stir in the remaining milk and the chocolate; cook over medium heat, stirring constantly, until the mixture begins to thicken. Reduce heat to low and simmer for 1 minute.

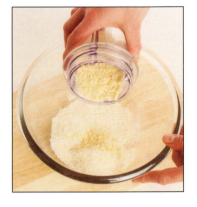

Remove from heat and stir in the vanilla. Pour into the pie shell. Chill for 2 hours. Serve with whipped cream (if desired).

Serves 8

Per serving: 243 Calories, Protein 5 g, Carb 23 g, Fiber 1 g, Total fat 15 g, Sat fat 4 g, Chol 5 mg, Sodium 32 mg
Exchanges: 0.7 Bread/Starch, 0.5 Other Carbs/Sugar, 2.8 Fat

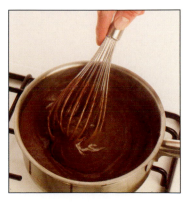

INDEX